More Than Pain Relief: The Essential Role of Palliative Care in South Africa

Mourine

First Printing, 2024

Contents

PART A: PROTOCOL

Background

South Africa (SA) is a middle-income country in the foot of the African continent, the second biggest economy in the region boosted by diverse economic activities[1] . However, there is inequity in distribution of health services[2]. SA health care system is funded mainly thorough a tax-generated funding. A recent SA burden of disease study revealed that there are four broad categories of disease or conditions that are the leading cause of morbidity and mortality in SA. These broad diseases categories include; communicable disease (excluding HIV and TB), TB and HIV, non-communicable diseases and injuries[3]. This disease burden puts strain on all components of health care; prevention, early detection, diagnoses, treatment, palliative care and survivorship (transition from treatment to extended survival)[4]. However, there is little investments on palliative care.

Palliative care is aimed at improving the quality of life of patients and their families who are facing problems associated with life-threatening illness, whether physical, psychosocial, or spiritual. The World Health Organization (WHO) defines palliative care as an approach that improves the quality of life of patients and their families facing the problem associated with life-threatening illness, through the relief of suffering by means of early identification and impeccable assessment and treatment of pain and symptoms, psychosocial and spiritual care[5]. For many years palliative care has been perceived as the act of giving pain medication to sufferers of life-threatening diseases but instead should be seen as promoting dignity, quality of life and adjustment to progressive illnesses, using the best available evidence. The rationale for palliative care certainly includes the need for relief from pain and other distressing symptoms, but it goes further to include efforts to enhance the quality of life, and even influence the course of illness in a positive way[6].

Patients in need of palliative care may require support from different levels of palliative care services during the course of their care, and it is important that there are referral pathways in place to ensure a seamless transition for patients and their families as well as providing these patients with quality and effective services[7, 8]. These categories of palliative care services are home based palliative care; mobile outreach services; outpatient care; inpatient palliative care facility; and consultative hospital based palliative care services from district level to tertiary hospitals. In a well-functioning system, there is a need for interaction and integration between these different levels of care[6, 9]

World Health Organization (WHO) recognised importance of palliative care, especially in low- and middle- income countries (LMICs), it has passed a resolution to strengthen palliative care during the 2014 World Health Assembly (WHA)[6, 7, 10]. Furthermore, it has been recognised that palliative care services have not been incorporated into the main health care services in the various levels of the health care system in many countries. This is an injustice to the sick, frail and weak who are suffering from life threating comorbidities, who without palliative care are often left to die in suffering without dignity and care. Despite palliative care being recognised as a crucial component of the health system, there have been very few studies establishing the cost component of Palliative care services (PCS) in South Africa for decision making.

This study will estimate the costs for consultative hospital based palliative care services (HBPCS). HBPCS are consultative services provided by a multidisciplinary palliative care team for inpatients. These services are provided through the following components of palliative care: identifying patients and continuity of care; symptom management; family support services; quality of life improvement; and end of life care. Each component has a requirement of resources, time and cost. In SA there is very limited generation of cost data relating to HBPCS. Due to improved life expectancy leading to an aging population in SA, it is expected that non-communicable diseases including cancer will raise. Therefore, – this increasing disease burden raises the need to integrate paliative care services ito the main health system services. This study will provide decision makers with cost components which can be used when integrating a palliative care services into an established tertiary hospital system.

Rationale

Palliative care services (PCS) maintain dignity and quality of life of sufferers. Health system reforms such as the re-engineering of primary health care (PHC) and introduction of National Health Insurance (NHI) aim to address the structural inequities of the health system and expand services coverage. The inclusion of PCS in the hospital-based services PHC is an essential move in responding to universal coverage which is a core concept of NHI. The need for PCS and palliative care education remains vital to contribute to the quality of life of patients, both adults and children in SA(11).

It is understandable that health care systems in LMICs are under increasing threat due to stagnant revenues and increasing health care demands due to communicable and non-communicable disease, injuries and other comorbidities. "Increasing access to palliative care services in low- and middle-income countries is often perceived as unaffordable despite the growing need of these services"(12), The South African Minister of Health, Dr Aaron Motswaledi, has demonstrated a commitment to PCS(13), but the pledge to make it work effectively must also come from varying levels within the Department of Health (DoH). An obstacle to overcoming this challenge is that palliative care as a health service has not been determined at all levels, currently there is no costing model in place(12). There are limited PCS costing studies that determines costs of all forms of palliative care services(12). This study aims to provide policy makers with the economic evidence to make optimal resource allocation decisions for HBPCS at a tertiary level in the Western Cape. This study will identify HBPCS, cost resources for this service and justify the funding requirements to sustain HBPCS in Groote Schuur Hospital (GSH).

Aim and Objectives

Aim

The aim of this study is to determine the costs and cost drivers for an existing hospital based consultative palliative care service (HBPCS) in South Africa adopting a providers' perspective.

Specific objectives

- To Identify and quantify resources needed in HBPCS in GSH
- To cost each category of quantified resource
- To develop a costing tool for HBPCS
- To estimate the cost per patient for providing a HBPCS in a tertiary hospital in South Africa
- To establish total operational cost for running HBPCS in a tertiary hospital in South Africa

Conceptual Framework

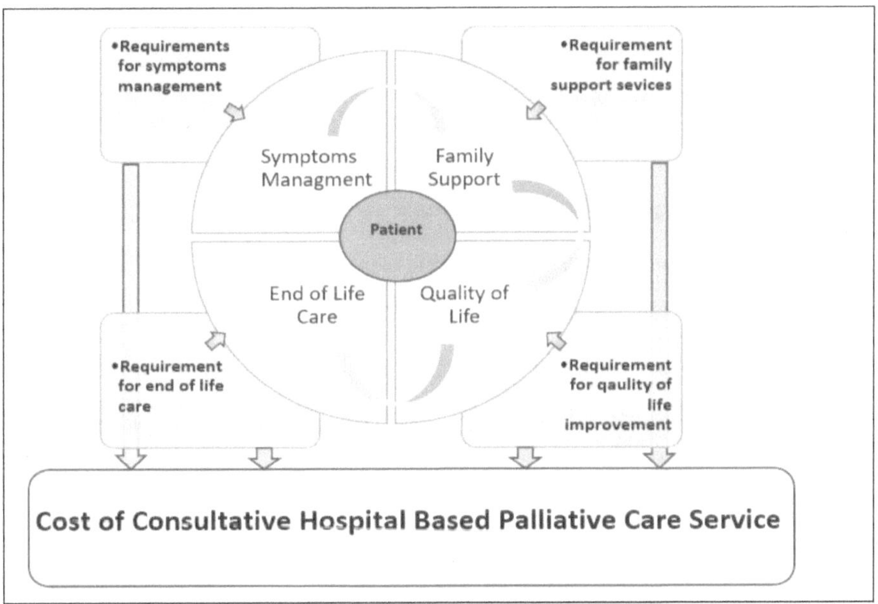

Figure 1: Conceptual Framework for costing HBPCS in Tertiary Hospital

Palliative care is well placed in the continuum of care detailed in the National Policy Framework and Strategy on Palliative Care (NPFSP) 2017-2022[13]. Palliative care services should be delivered by a multidisciplinary team that will provide care that is respectful and responsive to individual patient's preferences, needs and values and ensuring that patients values will guide clinical decisions. The aim and objectives of this study will be to identify resources required, quantify these resources and cost resources accordingly for HBPCS in a tertiary hospital. All costs will be added together to establish a total operational cost for running HBPCS in a tertiary hospital. This study will provide evidence that will be useful in informing resource allocations for integration of palliative care in the Western Cape. A palliative care patient is eligible for palliative care if they have been diagnosed with life threatening disease for which cure is not possible and require pain management, psychosocial care and spiritual care. Palliative care should not be seen only at the end of life in the disease trajectory, but it should be started together with curative care. The understanding is that the demand for palliative care will increase while the demand for curative care reduces over disease trajectory for patient diagnosed with life threatening diseases.

Proposed Study Design

This retrospective study will use a mixed method approach adopting a provider's perspective to measure the incremental cost of an existing public HBPCS in a tertiary hospital. This study will cost all inputs including recurrent and capital costs associated to the consultative palliative care services and in-kind contributions (labour and non-labour). A combination of inventory audits, interviews and observations will be used to collect the necessary data based on palliative care services. These costs will be projected over the 2018/19 fiscal year. An annual cost per patient will be calculated using the unit costs generated and number of visits per annum per patient. The expenditure and budget item allocations for HBPSC in GSH will be sourced from Western Cape (WC) Department of Health (DoH), any other data will be collected directly within GSH. This study will be conducted in collaboration with the palliative care team at GSH and the Western Cape DoH who are in the forefront in implementing palliative care services in the Western Cape.

Study ethical approval will be sought from the University of Cape Town Human Research Ethics Committee (HREC). Once ethical approval has been obtained researchers will start to develop a costing tool in Microsoft Excel. This tool will be developed in consultation with the palliative care team in GSH and the Western Cape DoH. It will account for all recurrent and capital costs incurred in the delivery of HBPCS in GSH. An inbuilt formulary will be incorporated into the tool to summarize costs. This costing tool will list inputs and detail quantities including prices associated with every input to estimate the unit cost per patient and the total cost of the service. This HBPCS tool will be validated and tested prior data collection in GSH to refine the tool. All costs will be in South African Rands (ZAR). A sensitivity analysis will be conducted to assess cost differences in the case where the HBPCS is delivered by a comprehensive multidisciplinary team. This sensitivity analyses will be used to estimate the changes in the cost of the PCS given a change in the size of the team. The findings of this study will be used to advocate for resources for PCS in tertiary level facilities both in GSH and the Western Cape province[14, 15].

Research Setting

This study will take place at GSH where the consultative HBPCS are already in place. GSH is one of the Western Cape's academic hospitals in Cape Town. The hospital is internationally renowned as the training ground for some of South Africa's doctors, surgeons and nurses[16]. GSH strives to provide outstanding tertiary care for patients of the Western Cape and beyond and has been one of the few facilities leading the implementation of PCS in the Western Cape. GSH is the only tertiary hospital in the Western Cape that provides a HBPCS. The patients seen by the palliative care team remain the responsibility of the admitting team (meaning that they remain the responsibility of the hospital ward in which they have been admitted), but are supported by the palliative care team through consultation for palliative care services[9]. Eligible patients are identified using the Palliative care assessment tool (Appendix 3).

Possible Difficulties and Solutions

It is understandable that some of the costing information will not be available at GSH. However, the Western Cape DoH should be able to provide researchers with actual and/ or estimates of cost information. Information on cost per personnel is considered confidential. Standard hourly rate for each pay class or category will be used to cost personnel instead of obtaining salary pay slips. All materials that are procured through the national government central supply database will be costed according to the actual purchase price listed in the central supply database understanding that these prices may differ from market prices.

Ethical Considerations

Ethical approval will be sought from the University of Cape Town Human Research Ethics Committee (HREC). This study will adhere to confidentiality, beneficence and non-maleficence considerations. All data that is collected will be stored safely and will only be accessed by researchers on this study. Anonymity will be maintained for all data regarding identity of staff and patients. There is no likelihood of any risks and dangers during this research study. Data on salaries will be reported by job title, patients seen in the study period will be head counted, these head counts will be used to estimate the average cost of care per patient. Researchers will use aggregated financial data, no pay slips, employee contracts, invoices or any proof of payments will be required, researchers do not foresee any harm for study participants, or anyone involved in the study.

References

1. IMF. World Economic Outlook: Growth Slowdown, Precarious Recovery. Washington, DC; 2018 April 2019.

2. Harris B, Goudge J, Ataguba JE, McIntyre D, Nxumalo N, Jikwana S, et al. Inequities in access to health care in South Africa. Journal of public health policy. 2011;32 Suppl 1:S102-23.
3. Pillay-van Wyk V, Msemburi W, Laubscher R, Dorrington RE, Groenewald P, Glass T, et al. Mortality trends and differentials in South Africa from 1997 to 2012: second National Burden of Disease Study. The Lancet Global Health. 2016;4(9):e642-e53.
4. Organization WH. World Health Report, 2010: health systems financing the path to universal coverage. World Health Report, 2010: health systems financing the path to universal coverage. 2010.
5. WHO Definition of Palliative Care: World Health Organization; 2016 [Available from: http://www.who.int/cancer/palliative/definition/en/.
6. WHO. Planning and implementing palliative care services: a guide for programme managers. 2016.
7. WHA67 R. 19. Strengthening of palliative care as a component of comprehensive care throughout the life course. Sixty-seventh World Health Assembly, Geneva. 2014;24.
8. Higginson IJ, Finlay IG, Goodwin DM, Hood K, Edwards AG, Cook A, et al. Is there evidence that palliative care teams alter end-of-life experiences of patients and their caregivers? Journal of pain and symptom management. 2003;25(2):150-68.
9. WHO. Planning and implementing palliative care services: a guide for programme managers.: World Health Organization; 2016.
10. Sasaki H, Bouesseau M-C, Marston J, Mori R. A scoping review of palliative care for children in low-and middle-income countries. BMC palliative care. 2017;16(1):60.
11. Rawlinson FM, Gwyther L, Kiyange F, Luyirika E, Meiring M, Downing J. The current situation in education and training of health-care professionals across Africa to optimise the delivery of palliative care for cancer patients. . ecancermedicalscience.8.
12. Hongoro C, Dinat N. A cost analysis of a hospital-based palliative care outreach program: implications for expanding public sector palliative care in South Africa. J Pain Symptom Manage. 2011;41(6):1015-24.
13. National Policy Framework and Stratergy on Palliative Care 2017-2022. In: DoH, editor. Pretoria: National Department of Health; 2017.
14. Ghabri S, Poullie AI, Autin E, Josselin JM. [HAS budget impact analysis guidelines: A new decision-making tool]. Sante publique (Vandoeuvre-les-Nancy, France). 2017;29(4):585-8.
15. Yagudina RI, Kulikov AU, Serpik VG, Ugrekhelidze DT. Concept of Combining Cost-Effectiveness Analysis and Budget Impact Analysis in Health Care Decision-Making. Value in health regional issues. 2017;13:61-6.
16. Cape Town South Africa: Western Cape Government [Available from: https://www.westerncape.gov.za/directories/facilities/823.

PART B: STRUCTURED LITERATURE REVIEW

Background

In many countries around the world, disease burdens continue to rise. This increase is attributable to improved life expectancy and many other factors which include socio economic conditions, unhealthy diets, sedentary lifestyles, and unhealthy behaviours[1]. In addition, advancement in technology as well as improved diagnostics and data reporting provide us with an opportunity to better observe and understand disease burdens. The burden of diseases refers to an epidemiological observation of diseases that describes mortality and morbidity of major diseases and risks factors to health. This observation can be at a global level, national level or district level[2, 3]. Health care systems in many countries are over stretched in response to increasing healthcare demand, resulting in a growing burden of communicable and non-communicable diseases. One of the main goals of healthcare is to cure diseases. However, a cure is not always possible, particularly in the current era of chronic diseases. In response to the need for comfort, relief from pain in chronic and life-threatening conditions for which cure is not feasible, palliative care emerged as an important consideration in healthcare[4]. The World Health Organization (WHO) defines palliative care as the prevention and relief of physical, psychological, social, or spiritual suffering experienced by patients living with life-threatening health conditions. It promotes dignity, quality of life and adjustment to progressive illnesses, using the best available evidence[5]. Palliative care has become a critical provision of health care especially in recent years due to life threatening conditions. With the current rate of observed burden of diseases, many people will be facing life-threatening diseases, injuries or life limiting health conditions and will require palliative care. Ideally, palliative care should be an important consideration for Universal Health Coverage and an essential service available to the whole population of a country without anyone suffering financial losses, neglect nor dying in seclusion. Despite this critical importance, very limited attention has been paid to palliative care globally.

In recent years, palliative care has been highlighted as an important consideration to be placed on the agenda for decision makers. However, the challenges of limited health care resources remain. In the 2014 World Health Assembly a resolution was adopted in which the WHO recommended that countries should facilitate the investment and integrate palliative care services in their respective health care systems[6]. However, in sub-Saharan Africa there is slow progress towards the inclusion of palliative care services. There are numerous factors hindering palliative care in every corner of the world, these include funding, availability of specialists and training[7]. The cost of proving palliative care at a population level has been one of the major barriers to access, particularly in resource-constrained settings. However, there are a limited number of economic evaluations and evidence around costing of palliative care services in Africa which makes it difficult for decision makers to estimate how much these services cost governments.

This literature review intends to map out and provide an insight into palliative care developments in Africa and describe factors influencing palliative care in this region. This analysis of the literature aims to identify studies describing costing approaches for palliative care interventions in sub-Saharan African countries and also to provide a brief evidence of the role of interest groups in achieving palliative care. Specifically, this review will aggregate evidence from relevant studies to provide an overview of costing considerations and costs for providing a palliative care in public hospitals in sub-Saharan Africa and in South Africa to be specific.

Domains of palliative care

Palliative can be delivered in one of the three main domains 1) home-based/ home care, 2) community-based, and 3) health facility based. Alternatively, these domains can be offered in combination of two or more simultaneously depending on affordability to the provider[8, 9]. These domains are described below:

Home-based/ home care palliative care services: These are the services provided in the home where patients live with their loved ones. They are best delivered by a trained palliative care team of health professionals. This approach is believed to be cost saving[10] in comparison to facility based palliative care models. In this approach of care family members are supported and trained in providing care, they are also integrated into the process and can facilitate referral to ancillary services, family members together with ward based outreach teams (WBOTs) ensure that their patient has easy access to care and their confidentiality and safekeeping is not compromised[11]. There are some disadvantages in providing home-based care palliative care services such as the difficulty in providing home-based care in situations where all family members are fulltime workers and, in such situations, they can even be compelled to forfeit their income to look after their loved ones. Chronic conditions can be costly or even impoverishing should conditions require that fulltime workers quit work to take care of their health or their loved ones.

Community-based services are sometimes referred to as hospice palliative care, are those offered by non-profit organisations, that are run by members of the community in local community health centres (CHC)[10]. These services require community participation, involvement, commitment, and dedication to be sustainable. They comprise community involvement in all levels, community-based palliative care services rely on voluntary funding, in-kind contributions and sometimes are financed by or on behalf of the patients. They can be run in poor or resource intensive community settings as long the public is committed to pledge or donate resources to run these services.

Health facility based palliative care services provide care for inpatients and outpatients. These services are rendered by trained palliative care professionals in health facilities such as clinics, hospitals and they sometimes require a multidisciplinary approach, specialists, and medical equipment to make the care more comprehensive. This approach of palliative care also facilitates a patient-centred approach which enables a smooth transition to care in the community and links patients to ward based outpatients teams (WBOT)[9, 10]. Effectiveness and intensity of care in these approaches has been studied in many settings. However, there is limited data on costing of these services, especially in the African region. Health facility based palliative care approaches can be classified as follows: outpatient palliative care clinic, hospital-based outreach palliative care, hospital-based consultative services, palliative care hospital day services and inpatient palliative unit. The palliative care clinic and the outpatient health facility based palliative care service reduces inpatient admissions which in turn reduces the provider costs but increases the rate of home deaths[(12)]. In contrast, treating patients in facilities is believed to increase the cost and the load for providers[(13)]. The consultative palliative care approach, where a palliative care multidisciplinary team of health professionals provide a consultative palliative care services to hospital inpatient admitted in different wards within the hospital is under studied with limited literature available.

The global landscape of palliative care

It was felt that palliative care was not getting the attention and the recognition from policy makers it that it required, and so there was an urgency to alert decision-makers, health professionals, and communities about the need of palliative care and its effectiveness[(14)]. This motivated many different concerned parties to join forces in various settings in the world to lobby for the integration of palliative care and for it to be considered as important as any other public health issue. One of the important initial steps was to conduct a study to assess the distribution of palliative care services around the world. Evidence provided by Wright et al. in 2008[(15)] mapped palliative care provision throughout the world (Figure 1), during this period palliative care was mostly provided in high income countries (HICs) with abundant health care resources. While the evidence revealed the need for palliative care services across many other countries.

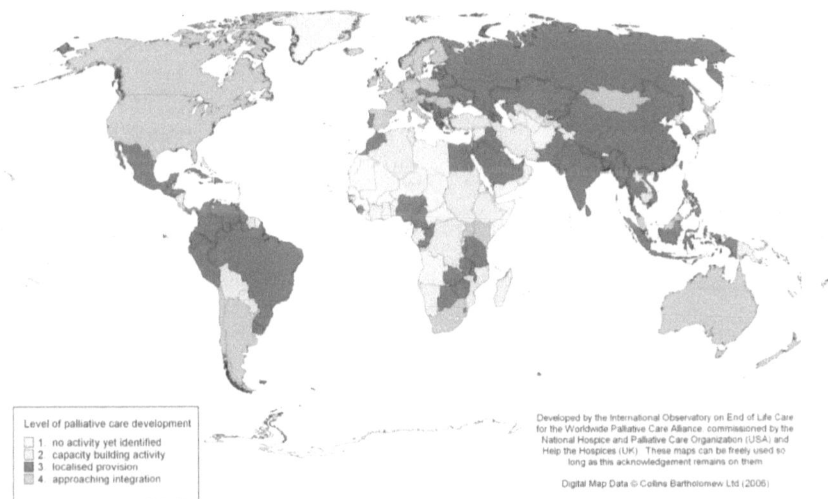

Figure 1: World map showing the level of palliative care development directly from Wright et al. 2008[(16)]

Wright et al. in 2008[(16)] categorized hospice-palliative care initiatives in different countries around the globe, these initiatives were represented in world and regional maps using a mathematical algorithms that involved the analysis of evidence from different sources; published and grey literature, regional experts, and a task force selected from palliative care advocacy bodies[(16)]. In this scoping review by Wright et al. palliative care interventions were identified in 115 of the total 234 countries originally included for study. The authors describe four categories that countries were assigned to, as follows: 1) 33% had no identified hospice-palliative care activity; 2) 18% had capacity building activities but no palliative care services; 3) 34% of countries had localized palliative care provision; and 4) 15% of countries had palliative care activities approaching integration with mainstream service providers[(16)].

This study showed disparities between LMICs and some of these were associated with the level of development of each country and the resources devoted to health care (especially for palliative care) in that country. Most of these palliative care interventions were provided by hospices, non-profit organizations, and the private sector. This study alone showed that palliative care awareness was needed to bring attention, recognition and commitment of decision makers and advocates to facilitate palliative integration especially in the public health sector of many countries. This study by Wright et al. in 2008[16] was performed more than a decade ago, and subsequently, an important report was published by the World Health Organization (WHO) in 2014 titled "Global Atlas of Palliative Care at the End of Life". This report updated and refined the estimates made by Wright et al. 2008[16]. According to this WHO report it is only 14% of the global population that has access to the highest standard of palliative care, and this access is more concentrated in European countries[17]. Due to these disparities, palliative care advocates rallied forces behind the agenda of integration of palliative care services and its recognition globally[14]. According to palliative care advocates, palliative care should include the dignity of the patient and the principles of urgency, universality and being non-discriminatory. The international palliative care community is supported by three prominent disciplines: palliative care, public health and human rights, in which specialists in these fields interact on an ongoing basis and over various platforms to achieve this common agenda. The international palliative care community argues that "...the care of the dying is a public health issue. Given that death is both inevitable and universal, the care of people with life-limiting illness stands equal to all other public health issues"[14]. Given the low number of articles sources, there is a need for updated studies to improve the available evidence.

The growing recognition of palliative care

Palliative care started as a religious institutional practice and it further evolved and was deemed important by caregivers to provide care for patients with terminal illnesses. In recent years we have seen how it has added value in patients with life limiting conditions. Palliative care has now been recognised as a human right[18]. This recognition was advocated by the global palliative care community on behalf of the weak and frail facing life limiting illnesses, who on their own cannot advocate for services they need. This achievement was realised after palliative care advocates, researchers and palliative care professionals around the world including Africa, joined forces to lobby for the realisation of palliative care and its recognition as a basic human right over many efforts in various platforms.

In 2002, the international community of palliative care drafted the Cape Town Declaration. This declaration articulated strategies, modalities, and essential principles to address the suffering related to life limiting conditions. This resolution endorsed palliative care as a basic human right for every patient facing a life limiting disease[19]. This was necessary because palliative care is essential and central to health and human dignity. Palliative care was endorsed for two reasons; 1) it does not foster or prevent death, but it provides effective response in alleviating suffering and pain ;2) it ensures that sufferers live active and pain free lives for as long they are alive. This resolution also endorsed availability of appropriate drugs such as opioids which was a challenge and limited in many African countries for many reasons, such as governments regulations put in place to avoid recreational use of opioids. Limited drug availability in many African countries can also be attributed to a low availability of specialist and doctors who are legally regulated to prescribing opioids in all levels of care. The lower levels of care are characterized by a sparse distribution of doctors making it difficult to access opioids in lower levels of care. For this reason, the resolution also endorses establishments of educational programmes for informal and formal providers of palliative care who are in the vanguard in delivering these services[19]. In short the resolution endorses the integration of palliative care in all levels of health care.

In 2005, the palliative care international community meet in Korea and drafted the Korean Declaration. The Korean Declaration[20] put emphasis on the major points articulated in the Cape Town declaration and further encouraged that all hospice and palliative care services should be included as part of all governmental health policy, as recommended by the WHO[6]. Further, in 2007 the international community drafted the Budapest Commitments[21]. The national associations of hospice and palliative care were developed further across regions and formulated what is known as the Worldwide Palliative Care Alliance (WPCA)[22]. While, pushing the same agenda over several mediums and platforms, WPCA supported the regional networks such as the International Association of Hospice and Palliative Care (IAHPC), the Asia-Pacific Hospice Palliative Care Association (APHPCA), the African Palliative Care Association (APCA), and the European Palliative Care Association (EPCA). These commitments called for extensive availability of patient centred and affordable palliative care services which are non-discriminatory. They further acknowledged that these services will be fostered through policies which will also consider primary health care principles. Lastly, these commitments acknowledged the lack of palliative care education and called for integration of palliative care education for informal education for caregivers and professional education for formal training of specialist. The biggest achievement of the forces behind WPCA was the World Health Assembly in 2014, where WHO recognised the worthiness of palliative care, especially in LMICs. In general, these resolutions aimed at fostering palliative care.

Scoping for this review

We consulted technical experts in the field of palliative care for their recommendation of several articles for inclusion in this study as a start set. Thereafter, a snowballing technique[(23)] for selecting relevant titles from the start set references list was undertaken. Formal literature review was done additional to the snowballing technique, articles were searched in various databases: Google Scholar, PubMed, and Scopus. For inclusion, studies were reviewed if they included any of the following terms: "palliative care", "development"," "initiatives", "goals", "Africa", "provider", "challenges", "end of life care", "opioids", "strengths" and "cost". The focus of this literature review was on studies conducted in low- and middle-income sub-Saharan African countries. Therefore, studies were deemed eligible only if they were palliative care studies that originated in Africa or were scoping reviews that included palliative care developments in the African continent. Using the snowballing technique was advantageous because we identified relevant papers and then used these article to drive the literature identification forward from reference lists of identified articles[(23)]. After the snowballing and database search, a total of 132 articles were identified. However, after thorough screening of these articles, we excluded 78 which were duplicates or were not relevant to this study and a total of 54 articles were found to be eligible for the structured literature review.

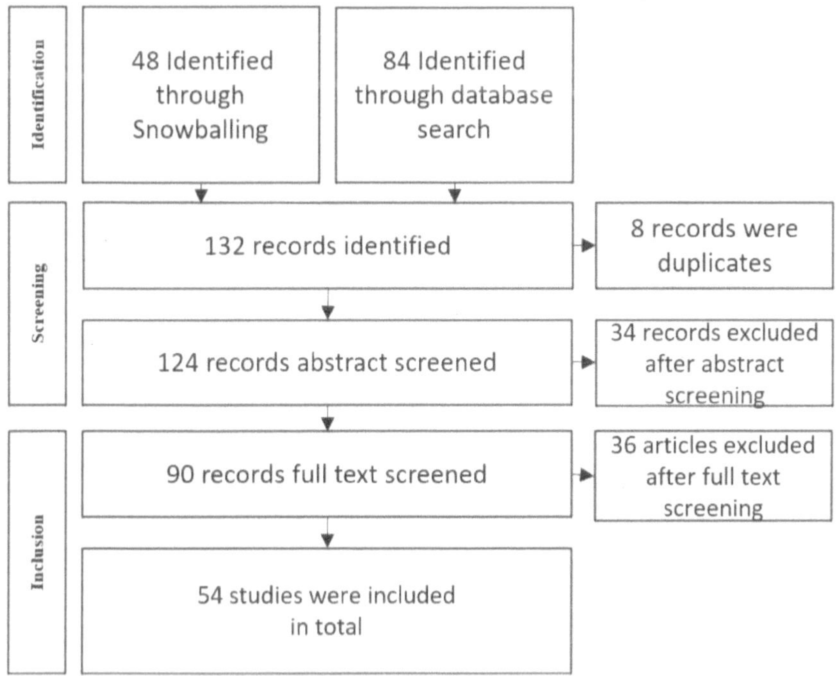

Figure 2: Preferred reporting items for systematic reviews and meta-analyses (PRISMA) Diagram

Palliative care services in Africa

A comprehensive scoping review study on palliative care was conducted between 2005-2016 for 26 African countries by Rhee et al. 2017[15]. This study assessed medical literature and included articles recommended by a local expert, published in four common languages. It sourced articles that articulated or mentioned: activities, policies, medicines, implementation, or advocates in palliative care. Selected articles had to meet a quality assessment criterion which was based on: 1) the journals impact factor, 2) journal ranking, 3) number of citations per article. There were 518 articles found (South Africa alone contributed a total of 210 articles) but only 49 of these articles met the quality and assessment criteria. Information on 26 (48%) of 54 African countries was found. Most services were concentrated in Kenya, South Africa, and Uganda, and 14 (26%) countries showed an increase in palliative care services during this timeframe. Stand-alone palliative care policies were existing in Malawi, Mozambique, Rwanda, Swaziland, Tanzania, and Zimbabwe. Postgraduate diplomas in palliative care were available in Kenya, South Africa, Uganda, and Tanzania[15]. Prescriber restriction laws, restrictions and access to opioids were identified as common barriers to adequate palliative care provision. Information on service provision and implementation was available for 19 countries with Kenyan, South Africa, Tanzania and Uganda and Zimbabwe with highest number or activities of palliative care services[15]. This study argued that "...availability of medicines remained a major issue across African countries, with access to morphine being a notable change, although opioid availability is not the only aspect of palliative care development"[15]. This study showed that information on palliative care development was concentrated on a subset of countries and that palliative care advocates should not only focus on scaling up services and medicines but should also focus on improving palliative care polices, education and research. It is important when evaluating palliative care to consider not just service provision, but focus be paid to; policies, implementation, drug availability such as opioids, education, interventions and services providers.

Palliative care services in Africa remain insufficient, there are a number of strategies that can be used to harness these services and facilitate greater service coverage[24] and palliative care services in the African region need to be enforced to address the rising demand placed by burden of diseases[25]. Two studies by Allsop and colleagues in 2018 and 2019[24, 25], argue that mobile Health (mHealth) interventions should be explored even further to archive wider coverage and access to palliative care for patients with life threatening conditions. These interventions include mobile phone applications, inbound and outboard call centres, and text messaging to educate or empower caregivers and patients with health education. Allsop et al. 2018, conducted a systematic review to identify the development and use of mHealth in palliative care services in sub-Saharan Africa. The authors plotted identified mHealth interventions against a modified WHO mHealth and information, communication and technology (ICT) framework to classify how they are targeting health system strengthening[24]. In total there were 110 articles identified, but only five of these articles met the inclusion criteria. These five articles describe mHealth interventions for palliative care services use in Nigeria, Uganda, Kenya and Malawi. However, there was no evidence of mHealth services in South Africa, which might be due to the lack of scientific documentation and publication relating to palliative care mHealth services. The second study by Allsop and colleagues in 2019, focused on the use of mHealth interventions in sub-Saharan Africa in reaching out to affected populations[25]. mHealth interventions are not a widespread model for provision of palliative care services and are under studied. Advancements in technology provides an appropriate opportunity to scale up provision of palliative care intervention such as mHealth and call centres to reach the marginalized population living in the outskirts of city centres. A full costing of these mHealth interventions would be useful to provide supplementary evidence for feasibility and decision making. However, palliative care models are under researched in their entirety.

Subsequently an online survey was conducted in 21 countries in the African continent to identify: current mHealth use in PC service delivery; potential barriers to mHealth use; and provider priorities for research development. There were 51 services identified throughout the region, only 74% of these services responded to the survey[23]. This online survey identified that there were barriers to mHealth which included "...not having access to phones, mobile network access, and limited access to expertise and hardware required for mHealth" and "...research priorities were identified which included exploring ways of incorporating mHealth into patient care and ensuring access and relevance of mHealth for patients and health professionals"[25]. Both these studies [15, 25] shows that mHealth palliative care services were present in Africa but so were barriers to accessing these services and that evidence-based mHealth interventions could form part of the evolving palliative care services in Africa[25]. The lack of basic infrastructure is notably the biggest challenge in exploring mHealth interventions in Africa.

The delivery of quality health care services is an important consideration of health care in any country. With the resolution of the WHO in 2014, palliative care has also been included as part of essential health services especially in low- and middle-income countries facing a quadruple disease burden of communicable and non-communicable diseases[(6)]. As we move to Universal Health Coverage the need to integrate palliative care services should be realized. Therefore, it will be necessary that all medical, social, and spiritual carers who forms part of the delivery of palliative care health services acquire the right skills to effectively deliver quality palliative care services that meet the needs of people facing life threatening conditions. A palliative care steering committee assembled in 2014 in Ireland developed a palliative care competency document[(26)]. This document aims to foster professional development of professionals who are in the forefront of the implementation of palliative care policies and identifies needs relating to these services. According to this document competences are generally a dynamic combination of knowledge, understanding, skills and abilities necessary to all palliative care teams. All of these are essential in any discipline however are especially important in palliative care service delivery. The only unfortunate part of this detailed competency framework was that it did not provide cost requirements for palliative care teams competencies.

Factors that influence palliative care development Africa

There are notable factors that enable advancement of palliative care. Conversely, there are also factors that hinder the advancement of palliative care. These factors may be different in different regions in the world, but they appear to be more remarkable in sub-Saharan African countries[(14)]. The ideas to introduce of Universal Health Coverage has provided an opportune moment to develop and integrate palliative care in the general health care services. The establishment and existence of advocating bodies and pioneering organizations have also played a role in achieving the development agenda of palliative care in many countries. Palliative care development refers to processes, structures, policies and resources that support the delivery of palliative care[(7)]. Rhee 2018 et al.[(14)]

described four factors (drivers, strengths, challenges and aspirations) influencing palliative care development in Africa.

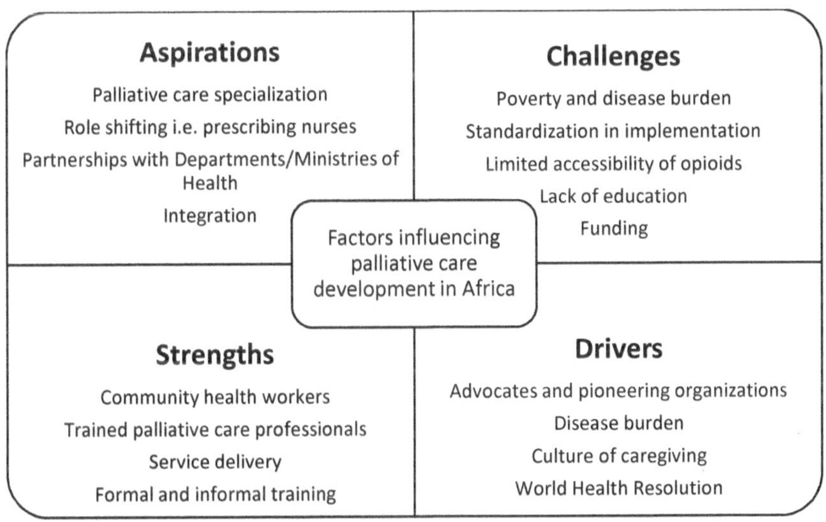

Figure 2: Factors affecting palliative care development: Adopted from Rhee 2018 et al.[7]

As indicated in Figure 3, 'strengths' refer to the factors that enable the implementation of palliative care services, they included workforce, diversity and the depth of services, research and palliative care education. These are inputs that are critical when delivering palliative care services for a population, they are mainly the building blocks of the actual services. In countries that already have plenty of these resources, structures and trained health care workers are more likely to succeed when implementing a palliative care service than countries with fewer of these inputs. Therefore, 'strengths' provide an enabling environment in rolling out and implementing a palliative care service. However, 'strengths' are more likely to be informed by 'drivers'.

'Drivers' refer to the activist and the pioneering organizations who mobilize, advocate and lobby for palliative care resources, policies and services. Often, 'drivers' meet to form alliances to add power to their voices and they set the agenda and put all their weight behind it. Countries with active activists and pioneering organizations are better off in terms of achieving palliative care expansions than those with passive advocates. Sometimes 'drivers' can be in the form of human forces and interactions behind certain policy agendas or shared goals such as efforts to combat diseases which pose risk and place burden on health systems like HIV/AIDS. Establishments that were formed to combat other diseases can also be used to achieve palliative care advancements and 'aspirations'.

'Aspirations' are the desires, hopes and ambitions to archive short- and long-term goals. The most prominent goal in palliative care is integration of palliative in all levels of health system. This goal was articulated in the World Health Assembly in 2014. However, 'aspirations' are more likely and easily attained when working in partnerships with other stakeholders. Partnerships ensures continuity and sustainability of health care services. A good example is when local non-profit organization are working hand in hand with government to provide holistic palliative care services such as when patients are discharged from tertiary or district hospitals that they can still access palliative care services within their communities and hospices. Having strong partnerships with all stakeholders (Department of Health, pioneering organizations and the private sector) also strengthens health services delivery. One of the most desired 'aspirations' in palliative care is permitting nurses to prescribe opioids for palliative care to allow patients to access drugs for symptom management at all levels of health care. However, more efforts are still needed to promote this idea especially in sub-Saharan African countries.

Very importantly, lack of availability of palliative care education; lack of standardization in implementation; limited availability or accessibility to pain management medication such as morphine and other opioids; poverty; disease burden and inadequate funding are persistent 'challenges' for many Africa countries[7]. Funding is required to ensure sustainability and to maximize existing resources to improve and expand services and infrastructure. Increasing access to palliative care services in African countries is often not a priority, even though people suffer, die in pain and with minimum effort invested into palliative care. There are a limited number of economic evaluations and costings of palliative care interventions and health care services in the African region generally. The lack of these economic evaluation for palliative care interventions creates a perception of unaffordability, this perception creates a disregard of palliative care services which further creates inequities in health care delivery especially for those patients who are suffering from life threatening conditions. Health care decisions should be based on: scientific evidence; use near real time clinical and costing data; and be based on patients values and preferences to improve transparency of reasoning behind policies that are aimed at improving quality of care, health care outcomes and treating all people with dignity[(27)].

There is an increasing demand for palliative care in sub-Saharan Africa, while access, availability and provision of services remains dubious and inadequately integrated into the national health services. In many African countries palliative care is largely reliant on missionary hospitals and non-profit organizations characterized by sporadic home-based care services. There are ongoing efforts to integrate palliative care into the general health services in these countries ever since the World Health Assembly in 2014. However, for integration to be successful there is a need to develop public health polices and public financing to sustain these programmes in Africa[(8)]. Furthermore, there is a need to invest in costing studies for palliative care in order to understand the cost component for providing these services. Costing studies for palliative care services can contribute greatly by providing information needed to make policy and program decisions.

Interest groups and their roles in achieving palliative care

In many developed and developing economies, aspirations to achieve palliative care have been driven successfully by interest groups (activist and pioneering organizations). In Kenya, the hospice association at the national level has lobbied, advocated and mobilized for the integration of palliative care[(28)]. The main aim was to ensure that all citizens who needed these services had access to palliative care close to their homes. The successful integration of palliative care has also resulted in: many health care professionals being trained in palliative care, integration of palliative care in public, private and mission health institutions and integration of palliative care in undergraduate medical and nursing studies[28]. Stakeholders involved in integrating palliative care were supportive throughout the levels of implementation as required. If Kenya has succeeded in integrating palliative care into the main health system, why would it be difficult to attain the realization of palliative care in South African. Many specialists and hospices in South Africa are members of the Hospice Palliative Care Association of South Africa (HPCA) which is also a member of the World Palliative Care Association[29]. Members of these alliances are advocates and come from various fields and specialization in palliative care such as academia and medicine. Therefore, they have the necessary power to drive the agenda, they are trained in palliative care service delivery and have the necessary experience in implementation and to incorporate palliative care education into the curriculum of various training institutions.

In Tanzania, there were several challenges in implementing the palliative care programme, these challenges were not unique, but common to other African countries[30]. They included limited accessibility to morphine (one of the common opioids used) and workforce. There were many lessons that were learned throughout the integration process in Tanzania. However, the main objective was achieved because there was a rapid scale up of palliative care services to individuals in poor settings, improved palliative care training for health care professional and there was an observed increase of patients receiving palliative care services. Going forward it would be useful for African countries to learn from the experience of other African countries that have rolled out palliative care programmes successfully. More economic evaluation studies and health impact analyses exercises are useful and should be undertaken to evaluate effectiveness of palliative care modalities in African countries.

Palliative care advocates are an important consideration in lobbying and mobilizing resources, especially when they are directly involved in agenda setting. They have the potential to assert pressure in the decision-making structures especially when they have one voice.

Accessibility and use of opioids in palliative care

Patients who are weak, frail and facing life-threatening illnesses often require opioids for pain, which is a common feature of palliative care[31]. Palliative care patients require clinical pain management through drugs such as opioids to; relieve pain; improve physical comfort; and enhance quality of life. Opioids targets the nervous system to reduce pain, they are commonly used in palliative care. In countries with intensive palliative care programmes there is large scale use of opioids. Equitable access to opioids is a major issue in many places in the world. About a quarter of the world's population (84.25%) lacks sufficient access to opioid drugs. More than 90% of global opioid intake was accounted for by Australia, Canada, New Zealand, the United States, and other European countries, while LMICs accounted for the remaining 10%[17]. . The many reasons that hinder opioids use include insufficient knowledge and training of medical professionals in pain management, fear that patients may become addicted, and legislative frameworks for control of opioids use in various countries. There are enormous challenges that are associated with morphine restrictions, distribution and use worldwide, these challenges present inequalities in the distribution of opioids between HICs and LMICs.

There are however countries that have archived a better rollout than others in Africa such as Uganda. Uganda has achieved a morphine roll-out programme in partnership with the palliative care interest groups in Uganda. A study was conducted in Uganda to evaluate the use of morphine for AIDS and cancer pain relief[32]. Researchers employed different data collection techniques in three phases to follow distribution of morphine and its use from production throughout the supply chain. These data collection techniques included interviews, observations, and clinical care audits in two palliative care facilities. Health care professionals, carers and government officials were interviewed to describe local prescribing guidelines, and morphine distribution was observed from entry into Uganda throughout pharmaceuticals and distribution into state hospitals, wards, and patients in their homes. While the clinical audits observed domiciliary nursing staff prescribing and issuing morphine for better access.

Results of the study shows that the model and the rollout of opioids offered a successful approach for patient care in Uganda. This study also tells us that advocates lobbied for relaxation of opioids regulation to improve accessibility and their use in which in turn benefitted palliative care patients allowing them to have quality life in their last days of life[33]. This model was a good reference case for other countries in Africa. Subsequent to this study we have seen many countries developing guidelines for opioids use South Africa being one of them. South Africa developed a guideline for opioids which aimed at assisting health care professional to screen, select, and initiate patients on pain management and further monitor and continue opioids use. These guidelines further took experience from other international guidelines[31, 34-36] to make it as comprehensive as possible. Today in South Africa pain management treatments can be prescribed from the Chronic Non Cancer Pain Guideline[37] or the WHO Model List of Essential Medicines[38]. The WHO guideline has a more comprehensive list. Countries can develop their own opioids guidelines and recommendations, and in their recommendation, they can use drugs that are effective but easily accessible and afforded. Opioids are an important feature in palliative care, they are being used to treat and relive chronic pain and they improve the quality of life of palliative care patients[37]. They are effective therapy in palliative care, their availability and use depict the quality of palliative care services in every setting, they can be used as indictors when monitoring palliative care services. Countries with eased opioids regulation are more likely to achieve better rollout and quality palliative care services.

Table 1. Opioids Recommended in South Africa taken directly from the Chronic Non Cancer Pain Guideline and WHO Model List of Essential Medicines[37, 38]

Recommendation for Chronic Non Cancer Pain Guideline	***Recommendation of the WHO Model List of Essential Medicines***
Buprenorphine Sublingual, transdermal	Acetylsalicylic acid
Fentanyl Transdermal	Ibuprofen
Hydromorphone Oral	Paracetamol
Morphine Oral	Codeine
Oxycodone Oral	Fentanyl
Codeine Oral	Morphine
Dihydrocodeine Oral	Methadone
Tramadol Oral	Amitriptyline
	Cyclizine
	Dexamethasone
	Diazepam
	Docusate sodium
	Fluoxetine a
	Haloperidol
	Hyoscine butyl bromide
	Hyoscine hydrobromide
	Lactulose
	Loperamide
	Metoclopramide
	Midazolam
	Ondansetron
	Senna

Palliative care as an essential component of health care in SA Palliative care services in South Africa require urgent consideration because of the demands that are being placed because of an ageing population and the disease profile found in the country. When people grow older in a population it is more likely that they suffer from non-communicable diseases and other chronic conditions. With these reasons among others palliative care should be an essential component of healthcare. Making palliative care a requirement for health care should include extending palliative care services to all eligible patients including people with non-cancer diagnoses. To determine whether palliative care should be an essential component of healthcare in South Africa, we have reviewed current evidence from the literature which we present here.

A study by Frankenfeld et al. 2019[39] found that 14.6% of all patients over the age of 18 years, that were admitted to 46 acute care public hospitals medical and surgical beds in the Western Cape Province of South Africa, died within one year of hospital admission. The mortality ratio was 1 in 5 of patients admitted to medical wards and almost 1 in 10 patients admitted to surgical beds die within one year. The greater percentage of deaths in patients admitted to medical beds was likely a reflection of the natural burden of disease in South Africa, with death predominantly due to both non-communicable and communicable diseases and this mortality was found to rise abruptly with age. This study revealed that patients admitted to specialised oncology beds, and those admitted to specialised tuberculosis hospitals had very high one-year mortalities of 50.8% and 29.9% respectively. This study used a Gold Standards Framework (GSF) prognostic indicator criterion[40, 41] for assessing palliative care need at a population level based on patient diagnoses and a retrospective approach of analysis of the one year post admission death registry data. The GSF tool criteria identified patients who are in their last year of life (retrospectively), it also assessed current and future (ahead in time while they are still alive), clinical and personal needs and plans across care in their final days.

The findings of this study reveal that there is a great need for palliative care in South Africa, 1570 (14%) of 10 761 patients admitted for acute care in 46 hospitals in Western Cape over a 2-week period in March 2012 died, also to take into consideration that this was just one of the nine provinces of South Africa, if the same methodology could be replicated in all provinces, we would likely see similar results. This was the first study in the African context providing this kind of evidence and it reveals that a high portion of patients who are admitted in the Western Cape acute care hospitals are in their final year of life. Another related assessment of palliative care need in South Africa provided similar findings[(42)]. Therefore, these findings suggest an investment into palliative care especially for those terminal disease condition such as cancer, TB and HIV based on need. Admission of patients into hospital may provide an opportune time to initiate palliative management for eligible patients. However, when they are discharged community WBOTs together with families can take over the management of these patients in the comfort of their homes.

Cost of providing palliative care services within the public sector of the South African health system

There was only one study that was identified in the sub-Saharan African region, this study was conducted in South Africa and it attempted to cost palliative care services in the public sector. The identified study used a gross costing approach which is known to have a poorer level of precision. In this study researchers attempted to measure the unit cost (cost per visit) for a hospital based outreach program[(13)]. In this study a total of 4493 and 3412 in hospital visits and outreach visits respectively were recorded. The costs per hospital outreach visit and in-hospital visit were R568 (US $71) and R640 (US $80) in 2011, respectively. This study found that hospital outreach services have a potential to avert hospital admissions in generally overcrowded services in low-resource settings and may improve the quality of life of patients in their home environments[(13)]. To our knowledge there has never been a study conducted in South Africa with a focus on costing other modalities of palliative care. While there are extensive costing and cost effectiveness study that we have seen in first world countries such as US, Canada, China and the United Kingdom. [(43-46)]. This gap highlights a need for further investments in research in palliative acre in the African continent. An important principle in Universal Health Coverage is ensuring that those needing care get to access the services they need whenever they need them. Specialists in palliative care understand that when rolling out a national comprehensive programme for palliative care these domains of 1) home-based/ home care, 2) community-based, 3) health facility based or 4) informal care can be delivered individually or in combination. So, investment into costing studies for these palliative care domains would help determine the cost of each and depending on the country's commitment to palliative care which domain could be affordable.

Integrating palliative care with community health workers programmes in South Africa

CHWs sometimes referred to WBOTs have been utilized in many countries to deliver outreach programmes such as: case finding, health education, home-based care, directly observed treatment strategies and other health services to patients in the comforts of their homes. These programmes have shown to have the potential to improve health outcomes in different settings and they have benefited those who are frail and living in areas that are difficult to access. An evaluation of CHWs investment for different health conditions was conducted in 2018 in South Africa for different diseases conditions such as: palliative care, HIV/AIDs, diabetes and hypertension and mother to child services. A South African Medical Research Council (SAMRC) working paper[10] reported the results of the investment case specifically looking at the costs and benefits in standard care scenario to a scenario of well performing CHWs platforms that are supported with adequate training, supervision, support and funding to achieve palliative care objective and other conditions. This study estimated that 1 out of 6 beds in the Cape Metropole alone are occupied by patients requiring palliative care and 50% of these patients are hospitalised for an average of two weeks. Therefore, when extrapolating to the population of the country the results shows if the 50% of the patients hospitalized were managed by WBOTs, 88 290 hospitalization would be avoided a year using the average hospitalization of two weeks. Daviaud et al.[10] further argues that for the same two weeks, palliative care at home would require one outreach visit by a doctor, an average of six visits by a professional nurse and eight visits by a community health worker. The yearly cost of home-based care, professional palliative clinicians and community health workers visits, would be R331 million, whilst it would have been R3.7 billion if managed in hospital. About R3.3 billion a year would be saved, or R29.3 billion over 10 years. There are however a number of assumptions made in this modelling. Such as patients requiring the same intensity of visits and that all patients would require a standard visit by a professional doctor over a defined period. Doctor led programmes are also more expensive than nurse led interventions. A full costing study for CHWs programme in palliative care would be very valuable. And it is important to remember that as much as the cost of providing the services is important the dignity provided to the patients and effectiveness of service is more important. There is no one better model of providing palliative care hence more of these models should be costed to provide costing data that can be used to determine what programmes are more effective when provided simultaneously in a comprehensive palliative care programme.

Important consideration when conducting a costing study in palliative care

It is very essential to examine the approaches that are used to generate data for estimating the cost of providing any services. There are various approaches in costing which include bottom up costing, top down costing and mixed approaches[27, 47]. The precision of these costing approaches varies, micro costing commonly known as a bottom-up approach have a higher level of precision and because of this high precision the findings of the study can be very accurate about the costs of a service. The micro costing approach follows a bottom-up costing technique and uses an ingredient approach to identify, quantify, and cost inputs for a service. Due to these reasons micro costing approaches are quite expensive in comparison to gross costing approaches, as they are resource intensive. Gross costing approaches have a poorer level of precision. The assumptions made in a gross costing may affect the accuracy of the cost estimate, as this as well as the reliability are highly dependent on the quality of secondary data[47]. For this reason, top-down costing studies are not appropriate measure of small changes in resource consumption. The gross costing approach follows a top-down costing technique, they can be easily conducted and are less expensive. Micro costing and gross costing approaches can also be used in combination to archive different objectives.

There are a very limited number of economic evaluations for palliative care domains (1) home-based/ home care, 2) community-based, or 3) health facility based Further research is required in this field to cost palliative care domains as discrete elements of care. These studies would produce cost evidence and frameworks that would reflect the full resource outlays and which can be adopted for future use[(48)]. It is imperative to have good costing data for palliative care interventions in order to inform decisions regarding resource allocations for palliative care services. Gardiner 2017 et al.[(48)], conducted a systematic review study to understand what resources (inputs), components are relevant for economic evolution of palliative care, in this systematic review study articles were selected based on distinct search terms followed by screening of abstract and screening of full articles. For this study, a total of 38 research papers met the inclusion criteria. However, only eight studies were finally included in the analysis. This review summarised studies to explicitly group components of cost according to type of costs and domain of palliative care. Table 2 below presents a summary of inputs costs for different domains of palliative care. This framework is helpful to guide researchers about types of resources and components for costing palliative care domains.

Table 2: Framework by Gardiner et al. outlining types of costs for different palliative care domains[48]

Palliative care domain	Types of costs
Health facility based - Hospital	Inpatient hospital admissions/bed days Personnel costs Medical supplies, equipment and aids, etc. Inpatient procedures (surgery, chemotherapy, etc.) Investigations, laboratory and diagnostic costs Drugs and medications Outpatient hospital admissions Emergency room visits Ambulatory costs and transport Hospital day care Outpatient procedures (chemotherapy, etc.) Chinese and herbal medicines Overhead costs (building costs and capital depreciation) Palliative care unit admission Palliative care outpatient clinics Palliative care consultative service
Home-based/ home care OR Community-based	General practitioner/family physician surgery visits Medical and nursing home visits (general practitioner, etc.) Allied health home visits (physiotherapy, occupational therapy, mental health) Other home visits (social services, home care, other careers) Drugs and medications Medical equipment, aids and adaptations Day care services Transportation Stays in long-term care facilities, care homes, nursing homes, skilled nursing facilities Transportation Diagnostic tests, laboratory costs Personal support (bathing, feeding, dressing, home help) Other social services (meals on wheels, etc.) Nutritional counselling Dental services Communication costs Residential respite care and rehabilitation Overhead costs Direct payments made to users so they can 'buy' their own services

Continued

Palliative Care Domain	Types of costs
Hospice and specialist palliative care	Inpatient hospice stays/bed days Personnel costs Medical supplies Inpatient procedures Investigations, laboratory and diagnostic costs Drugs and medications Equipment and aids Outpatient appointments and clinics Home hospice Home visits from specialist palliative care Start-up costs, e.g., for new community palliative care nursing service
Informal care	Home caregivers Household help Equipment, aids, home adaptations Medications Insurance payments Travel and accommodation expenses Out-of-pocket expenses (parking, food/drink) Income lost from work Caregiver time costs Co-payments, e.g., shared with insurer/other

The Gardiner et al.[48] study is important in guiding health economists who conduct costing for palliative care interventions, as it explicitly describes inputs that should be considered and that are relevant for different domains of palliative care programmes. The results suggest a framework for identifying inputs that can be considered in three key domains of palliative care: (1) home-based/ home care, 2) community-based, or 3) health facility and further emphasized that the most important decision to make when conducting a costing study is deciding which perspective to adopt[48]. There are generally three perspectives to adopt when conducting a costing study:1) public provider perspective, in this perspective the state uses effective financing mechanisms to pool funds and use these funds to purchase services on behalf of the population. 2) the individual or household perspective, in this approach the patients or their households bears the cost of consuming the services and 3) the societal perspective, in this approach all actors in the production and consumption of service bears the cost of the services. These choice can mean a lot in the analysis of the costs and can have a great influence in decision making[49].

Considerations for ensuring quality and accuracy for a costing study

Costing studies like any research study must ensure that the findings are accurate and are of high quality. It is the aim of every researcher to produce cost estimates that are close to reality. In costing all identified resources utilised should be quantified and costed. To produce a quality costing output requires researchers to access several provider and patients' records. In addition, seeking the opinion of experts, health professionals and the patients as well as the carers is very useful. These experts are specialist and agents in the policy implementation and their experience is useful in guiding researchers to develop a costing framework. In the study methodology section of the proposed study, we have indicated that service provider such as nurses, auxiliary workers and doctors who work in the palliative care service will be interviewed and will assist researchers in the identification and costing of all resources. According to Yazback 2001[50] to consider very importantly methodological issues such as measurement techniques, costing perspective and time horizon in order not to deviate from costing principles. Researchers need to carefully construct and identify clear aims and objectives of the costing study, this is very helpful in constructing realistic questions that will guide researchers to achieve the research objectives in a more answerable and measurable manner.

The selection of the methodology should match the objectives of the study. It should be indicated clearly in the study the suitability of the methodology for calculating associated costs. The selected methodology should be able to identify and quantify all resources to establish a cost for the programme. The study should adopt a perspective of the costing procedure to have a clear understand of who is bearing these costs. The time period for the costing analysis should be clearly defined and be realistic, if costs are converted the conversion of currency should be clear, and amortization of resources that have a life expectancy of more than one year should be accounted for. Researchers need to use a tested or a realistic data collection tool, the data collection tool should account for recurrent and capital costs and should aspects of these not be accounted for then there should be a tangible reasoning as to why. The costing study should try as much as possible to take advantage of all data sources, so that the findings and results can be as close to the truth as possible. If any assumption is made, it should be stated explicitly so that everything is clear to the reader. Sensitivity analyses should be conducted to test robustness of assumptions and the findings should be presented very clear.

Conclusion

Literature suggest that palliative care services are widely adopted in developed countries, while they are significantly lagging in low resource countries. It has been estimated that inpatient services alone are available in about two-thirds of all hospitals in developed countries[51]. Research in developed countries has demonstrated improved quality of life for palliative inpatients for symptom control and satisfaction with care[52]. Due to these inpatient palliative care services families have benefited from emotional support, care planning and transitions of care. The outcomes of palliative care services including reduced hospital length of stay, hospital costs, and improved discharge status. Palliative care services have the ability to improve quality of life and avert hospital admissions[13]. While palliative care for patients hospitalized with advanced disease results in lower costs of care and less utilization of intensive care[53, 54]. However, there is scant literature on direct comparison on cost effectiveness of these palliative care domains or modalities. These domains are complimentary to each other, however when offered in combination they would be very resource intensive and unaffordable to low-income countries. In addition, there is no single domain that has been proven to be more effective than the others. Research is required to provide costing models for palliative care in general and to support such evidence with effectiveness of palliative care programmes in conjunction with cost of providing these services. Palliative care is under-researched in Africa and due to the demand placed on health care system more cost evidence in implementing palliative care is needed.

Sub-Saharan Africa, in a setting of scarce resources and high disease prevalence will need to scale up palliative care services and integrate palliative care into the general health services. Palliative care services are essential especially to those facing life threatening disease conditions, and yet there are very few studies that has been done in sub-Saharan Africa to show how to incorporate these services in public health care systems. Instead palliative care services are perceived as costly and unaffordable even though there is very limited literature around their costs, which can be a barrier especially in decision making[27]. Palliative care is in its infancy in Africa, there are attempts to drive the palliative care agenda in South Africa, especially around palliative care education, advocacy and drug availability. However, South Africa is lagging in terms of funding, standardizing and integration of palliative care services within the general health care in the country. Challenges associated with palliative care development are common in many African countries and they include: lack of funding; education; lack of standardization in implementation; reduced access to and availability of morphine, poverty and disease burden. In a country with influential advocates and advocacy groups some of these challenges can be addressed.

In conclusion, during the time of this review there was only one study that identified full cost of hospital based palliative care services in the public sector in sub Saharan Africa[13]. Many studies at end-of-life care in this region focused rather on costing specific disease conditions which do not reflect the full cost of palliative care services. We have seen middle income and higher income countries outside of the sub-Saharan region conducting full economic evaluations mainly for three palliative care domains[55-57], countries with health economics as an established discipline such as Canada, Turkey and Hong Kong having more robust studies in this filed. Insufficient costing evidence in the African region makes it even difficult for decision makers to even consider palliative care. However, this lack of cost data highlights the need for the proposed study which will assess a consultative palliative care model in a tertiary hospital.

References

1. Global, regional, and national incidence, prevalence, and years lived with disability for 354 diseases and injuries for 195 countries and territories, 1990-2017: a systematic analysis for the Global Burden of Disease Study 2017. Lancet. 2018;392(10159):1789-858.
2. Pillay-van Wyk V, Msemburi W, Laubscher R, Dorrington RE, Groenewald P, Glass T, et al. Mortality trends and differentials in South Africa from 1997 to 2012: second National Burden of Disease Study. The Lancet Global Health. 2016;4(9):e642-e53.
3. Abubakar I, Tillmann T, Banerjee A. Global, regional, and national age-sex specific all-cause and cause-specific mortality for 240 causes of death, 1990-2013: a systematic analysis for the Global Burden of Disease Study 2013. Lancet. 2015;385(9963):117-71.
4. Abdulaziz A, Zahid A. Palliative care: Time for action. Oman Medical Journal. 2016;31(3):161-3.
5. WHO Definition of Palliative Care: World Health Organization; 2016 [Available from: http://www.who.int/cancer/palliative/definition/en/.
6. WHA67 R. 19. Strengthening of palliative care as a component of comprehensive care throughout the life course. 2014.
7. Rhee JY, Garralda E, Namisango E, Luyirika E, de Lima L, Powell RA, et al. Factors Affecting Palliative Care Development in Africa: In-Country Experts' Perceptions in Seven Countries. Journal of pain and symptom management. 2018;55(5):1313-20.e2.
8. Mwangi-Powell FN, Powell RA, Harding R. Models of delivering palliative and end-of-life care in sub-Saharan Africa: a narrative review of the evidence. Curr Opin Support Palliat Care. 2013;7(2):223-8.
9. WHO. Planning and implementing palliative care services: a guide for programme managers. 2016.
10. Daviaud E, Besada D, Budlender D, Sanders D, Kerber K. Saving lives, saving costs: investment case for community health workers in South Africa. Cape Town: South African Medical Research Council. 2018.
11. Downing J, Powell RA, Mwangi-Powell F. Home-Based Palliative Care in sub-Saharan Africa. Home Healthcare Now. 2010;28(5):298-307.
12. Desrosiers T, Cupido C, Pitout E, van Niekerk L, Badri M, Gwyther L, et al. A hospital-based palliative care service for patients with advanced organ failure in sub-Saharan Africa reduces admissions and increases home death rates. J Pain Symptom Manage. 2014;47(4):786-92.
13. Hongoro C, Dinat N. A cost analysis of a hospital-based palliative care outreach program: implications for expanding public sector palliative care in South Africa. J Pain Symptom Manage. 2011;41(6):1015-24.
14. Gwyther L, Brennan F, Harding R. Advancing palliative care as a human right. Journal of pain and symptom management. 2009;38(5):767-74.
15. Rhee JY, Garralda E, Torrado C, Blanco S, Ayala I, Namisango E, et al. Palliative care in Africa: a scoping review from 2005-16. The Lancet Oncology. 2017;18(9):e522-e31.
16. Wright M, Wood J, Lynch T, Clark D. Mapping levels of palliative care development: a global view. J Pain Symptom Manage. 2008;35(5):469-85.
17. Connor SR. Global Atlas of Pallitiave Care. World Health Organization; 2020.
18. Gwyther L, Brennan F, Harding R. Advancing palliative care as a human right. J Pain Symptom Manage. 2009;38(5):767-74.
19. Mpanga Sebuyira L, Mwangi-Powell F, Pereira J, Spence C. The Cape Town Palliative Care Declaration: home-grown solutions for sub-Saharan Africa. J Palliat Med. 2003;6(3):341-3.
20. NHPCA. The Korea declaration Report of the second global summit of National Hospice and Palliative Care Associations, Seoul, Korea. Korea: National Hospice and Palliative Care Associations.; 2005.
21. EAPC. The Budapest Commitments European Association for Palliative Care; 2007.

22. Praill D, Pahl N. The worldwide palliative care alliance: networking national associations. J Pain Symptom Manage. 2007;33(5):506-8.
23. Wohlin C, editor Guidelines for snowballing in systematic literature studies and a replication in software engineering. Proceedings of the 18th international conference on evaluation and assessment in software engineering; 2014: Citeseer.
24. Allsop MJ, Powell RA, Namisango E. The state of mHealth development and use by palliative care services in sub-Saharan Africa: a systematic review of the literature. BMJ Support Palliat Care. 2018;8(2):155-63.
25. Allsop MJ, Namisango E, Powell RA. A survey of mobile phone use in the provision of palliative care services in the African region and priorities for future development. J Telemed Telecare. 2019;25(4):230-40.
26. Ryan K, Connolly M, Charnley K, Ainscough A, Crinion J, Hayden C, et al. Palliative care competence framework 2014: Health Service Executive (HSE); 2014.
27. Drumond, Michael, Schulpher M, George W, Torrence, O'Brien B, Stodddart G. Methods for the Economic Evaluation of Health Care Programmes 3rd Edition2005.
28. Ali Z. Integrating Palliative Care in Cancer Care in Kenya. Journal of Global Oncology. 2018;4(Supplement 2):164s-s.
29. HPCA. Annual Report. Hospice Palliatiev Care Association of South Africa 2019.
30. Nanney E, Smith S, Hartwig K, Mmbando P. Scaling up palliative care services in rural Tanzania. Journal of pain and symptom management. 2010;40(1):15-8.
31. Furlan AD, Reardon R, Weppler C. Opioids for chronic noncancer pain: a new Canadian practice guideline. Cmaj. 2010;182(9):923-30.
32. Logie DE, Harding R. An evaluation of a morphine public health programme for cancer and AIDS pain relief in Sub-Saharan Africa. BMC public Health. 2005;5(1):82.
33. Staff WHO, Organization WH. Cancer pain relief: with a guide to opioid availability: World Health Organization; 1996.
34. Raphael J, Ahmedzai S, Hester J, Urch C, Barrie J, Williams J, et al. Cancer pain: part 1: Pathophysiology; oncological, pharmacological, and psychological treatments: a perspective from the British Pain Society endorsed by the UK Association of Palliative Medicine and the Royal College of General Practitioners. Pain medicine. 2010;11(5):742-64.
35. Chou R, Fanciullo GJ, Fine PG, Adler JA, Ballantyne JC, Davies P, et al. Clinical guidelines for the use of chronic opioid therapy in chronic noncancer pain. The Journal of Pain. 2009;10(2):113-30. e22.
36. Manchikanti L, Abdi S, Atluri S, Balog CC, Benyamin RM, Boswell MV, et al. American Society of Interventional Pain Physicians (ASIPP) guidelines for responsible opioid prescribing in chronic non-cancer pain: Part 2--guidance. Pain physician. 2012;15(3 Suppl).
37. Raff M, Crosier J, Eppel S, Meyer H, Sarembock B, Webb D. South African guideline for the use of chronic opioid therapy for chronic non-cancer pain. South African Medical Journal. 2014;104(1):79-89.
38. Organization WH. World Health Organization model list of essential medicines: 21st list 2019. World Health Organization; 2019.
39. Frankenfeld P NvL, Manning K, Tiffin N, Raubenheimer P.J. One year mortality after hospital admission as an indicator of palliative care need in South Africa: incident cohort study 2019.
40. Gott M, Frey R, Raphael D, O'Callaghan A, Robinson J, Boyd M. Palliative care need and management in the acute hospital setting: a census of one New Zealand Hospital. BMC Palliat Care. 2013;12:15.
41. Thomas K, Wilson JA, Team G. Prognostic indicator guidance (PIG). The gold standards framework centre in end of life care CIC. 2011.
42. van Niekerk L, Raubenheimer PJ. A point-prevalence survey of public hospital inpatients with palliative care needs in Cape Town, South Africa. S Afr Med J. 2014;104(2):138-41.

43. Smith S, Brick A, O'Hara S, Normand C. Evidence on the cost and cost-effectiveness of palliative care: a literature review. Palliative medicine. 2014;28(2):130-50.
44. Pham B, Krahn M. End-of-Life Care Interventions: An Economic Analysis. Ontario health technology assessment series. 2014;14(18):1-70.
45. Hsu YC, Chu FY, Chen TJ, Chou LF, Chang HT, Lin MH, et al. Lots of little ones: Analysis of charitable donations to a hospice and palliative care unit in Taiwan. Int J Health Plann Manage. 2019;34(4):e1810-e9.
46. Coyle D, Small N, Ashworth A, Hennessy S, Jenkins-Clarke S. Costs of palliative care in the community, in hospitals and in hospices in the UK. Critical reviews in oncology/hematology. 1999;32(2):71-85.
47. Mogyorosy Z, Smith P. The main methodological issues in costing health care services: a literature review. 2005.
48. Gardiner C, Ingleton C, Ryan T, Ward S, Gott M. What cost components are relevant for economic evaluations of palliative care, and what approaches are used to measure these costs? A systematic review. Palliative medicine. 2017;31(4):323-37.
49. Dewa CS, Trojanowski L, Cheng C, Hoch JS. Potential effects of the choice of costing perspective on cost estimates: An example based on 6 early psychosis intervention programs. The Canadian Journal of Psychiatry. 2016;61(8):471-9.
50. Yazbeck A. Making Costing Fun! PowerPoint presentation, at the session entitled "How Much Does it Cost?" in the WBI's Adjusting to Change Learning Program Core Course on Population. Reproductive Health and Health Sector Reform World Bank, Washington, USA. 2001.
51. Liu OY, Malmstrom T, Burhanna P, Rodin MB. The evolution of an inpatient palliative care consultation service in an urban teaching hospital. American Journal of Hospice and Palliative Medicine®. 2017;34(1):47-52.
52. El-Jawahri A, Greer JA, Temel JS. Does palliative care improve outcomes for patients with incurable illness? A review of the evidence. Database of Abstracts of Reviews of Effects (DARE): Quality-assessed Reviews [Internet]: Centre for Reviews and Dissemination (UK); 2011.
53. Penrod JD, Deb P, Dellenbaugh C, Burgess JF, Jr., Zhu CW, Christiansen CL, et al. Hospital-based palliative care consultation: effects on hospital cost. Journal of palliative medicine. 2010;13(8):973-9.
54. Penrod JD, Deb P, Luhrs C, Dellenbaugh C, Zhu CW, Hochman T, et al. Cost and utilization outcomes of patients receiving hospital-based palliative care consultation. Journal of palliative medicine. 2006;9(4):855-60.
55. Saygili M, Çelik Y. An evaluation of the cost-effectiveness of the different palliative care models available to cancer patients in Turkey. Eur J Cancer Care (Engl). 2019;28(5):e13110.
56. Klinger CA, Howell D, Marshall D, Zakus D, Brazil K, Deber RB. Resource utilization and cost analyses of home-based palliative care service provision: the Niagara West End-of-Life Shared-Care Project. Palliat Med. 2013;27(2):115-22.
57. Wong FKY, So C, Ng AYM, Lam PT, Ng JSC, Ng NHY, et al. Cost-effectiveness of a transitional home-based palliative care program for patients with end-stage heart failure. Palliat Med. 2018;32(2):476-84.

PART C: MANUSCRIPT

MANUSCRIPT

Background

The Sub-Saharan African region has sparse palliative care established to cater for patients facing life limiting conditions. In South Africa, costing frameworks for palliative care interventions for the public sector do not exist and the cost of running a comprehensive palliative care programme remains unknown. There are few costing studies to inform costs of palliative care models which are necessary for decision makers to base their decisions on. The aim of this study was to determine the costs and cost drivers for hospital based consultative palliative care service (HBPCS) in South Africa adopting a providers' perspective.

Methods

In this empirical costing study, we developed and utilised a costing tool that employed a mixed bottom-up and top-down costing method to estimate the incremental cost of an existing hospital based consultative palliative care services (HBCPCS) in a tertiary hospital in Cape Town, South Africa, called Groote Schuur Hospital (GSH) adopting a public provider perspective. All inputs where valued using bottom-up, ingredients-based methods, except for direct staff where a top-down approach was utilised to allocate the staff's full salary to palliative care services. We collected costing data by conducting inventory audits, key informant interviews and observations. All inputs required in the production of the HBCPCS were checked against a costing framework for economic evaluations of palliative care interventions to ensure that the cost estimates were as inclusive as possible. All inputs with a lifespan of more than one year were annuitized using a 3% rate.

Results

The total annual cost for running the HBCPCS was R2 494 419 including both recurrent and capital costs. Recurrent items alone accounted for 96% (R2 392 407). While capital items accounted for 4% (R102 013) during the study period. The total cost per visit was R642 including the standard drug treatment package (R16). The major cost driver in the service was personnel accounting or 91% of the total annual cost. While a scenario analysis shows that when the size of the team size is doubled then the cost of direct personnel would increase to R4.4 million.

Conclusion

We have estimated the incremental unit cost of HBCPCS to be R642 per visit, the major cost driver being personnel. If funding allows, with an annual cost of R2.4 million these services can be provided in a public tertiary hospital as an adjunct to inpatient care for patients as a strategy for integrating palliative care to general health care services, as has been done at GSH. The HBCPCS was less costly when compared to hospital-based outreach palliative care programmes.

MANUSCRIPT TITLE PAGE

TITLE: The cost of providing consultative palliative care services in a tertiary hospital setting

1. Health Economics Unit and Division, School of Public Health and Family Medicine, Faculty of Health Sciences, University of Cape Town.
2. Department of Family Medicine, School of Public Health and Family Medicine, Faculty of Health Sciences, University of Cape Town.
3. Cancer Research Initiative, Deans Office, Faculty of Health Sciences, University of Cape Town.
4. Women's Health Research Unit, School of Public Health and Family Medicine, Faculty of Health Sciences, University of Cape Town.
5. South African Medical Research Council Gynaecology Cancer Research Centre, Faculty of Health Sciences, University of Cape Town.

Keywords: Palliative care, cost analysis, hospital-based services, cost, sustainability, hospital, costing framework, advocacy.

Introduction

In recent years we have seen a growing recognition of palliative care services in many regions of the world. However, in low- and middle-income countries there is limited data on access, availability, and utilization of palliative care interventions[1-3]. This lack of evidence hinders the design and implementation of effective policies and health services that would serve palliative care patients[4]. Palliative care has not been equitably integrated and funded like other health services, especially in Africa. It is now more than five years since the 67th World Health Assembly (WHA) where the World Health Organization (WHO) passed a resolution for governments to integrate palliative care services into the main health care services in their respective countries[5]. South Africa published a National Policy Framework and Strategy on Palliative Care for the period 2017-2022, this strategy has demonstrated a commitment to palliative care. However, palliative care has not yet been integrated as per the WHO recommendation in South Africa[6]. Furthermore, the burden of disease in South Africa makes it impossible to overlook palliative care services in the country[7, 8]. Many patients continue to be discharged into the care of their families who are often not provided with the necessary support. This can result in patients not receiving the care they may need and places additional financial burden on families.

The introduction of Universal Health Coverage (UHC) presents an ideal opportunity to redress and strengthen palliative care services in South Africa. Universal access for palliative care services continues to be scantily available and is often only a commodity of the wealthier in society. Across many African countries there are challenges and opportunities for the development of palliative care. Factors that augur well for the delivery of these services within the African region include the caregiving nature of communities, experience in dealing with chronic conditions such as tuberculosis (TB) and human immunodeficiency virus (HIV) and for some countries reasonably performing health care systems. However, adequate funding has been perceived as the major challenge that impedes the integration of palliative care[9, 10].

In South Africa deaths from non-communicable diseases increased progressively from 1997 to 2012 and the top ten causes of mortality have not changed during this period[8]. WHO mortality statistics reveal that non-communicable diseases are the leading cause of the deaths in South Africa, the broad cause of death by age shows that this disease category alone contribute up 65.77% to 67.82% for the age groups 55-74 and above 75 respectively which is a rate of 399.5 per 100 000 population for non-communicable diseases in the period 2015-2019[11]. In the Western Cape Province alone the mortality ratio due to non-communicable diseases and HIV was 1 in 5 patients admitted to medical wards and almost 1 in 10 patients admitted to surgical beds, with most patients dying within one year following their admission[12]. The top mortality trends in the Western Cape Province are similar to the national disease profile in South Africa[12]. The four disease categories that require palliative care most frequently are malignant neoplasms (28.2%), HIV diseases (22.2%) , cerebrovascular diseases (14.1%), dementias (12.2%)[13]. Jointly the other conditions make up the remaining 23.3%[13]. These statistics show a great need for palliative care interventions for the general population and especially for those patients who suffer from life limiting illnesses[12, 14]. Palliative care aims to prevent and relieve pain and other distressing symptoms by means of impeccable assessment and management within a team which includes the patient's family[15] The palliative care approach also integrates psychological and spiritual aspects of patient care, and very importantly a specialist provides support to the family during the patient's illness and in bereavement. There is a perception of unaffordability, despite a lack of economic evaluation evidence for palliative care interventions. This can create a disregard of palliative care services which further creates inequities in health care delivery especially for those patients who are suffering from life limiting conditions.

Costing frameworks for palliative care interventions for the public sector in South Africa do not exist and the cost of running a comprehensive palliative care programme remains unknown. However, we have consulted guidelines such as the Global Health Cost Consortium Reference Case[16] to guide our cost estimation. To date there has not been much investment in performing costing studies in South Africa to assess the few palliative care domains being practised even during this window period of introduction of UHC in the country. We have only found one costing study undertaken for a hospital based outreach service in palliative care for a public provider[17], while other domains have not had published cost analyses. The aim of this study is to establish the incremental costs for hospital based consultative palliative care service (HBCPCS) in a tertiary facility in Cape Town, South Africa adopting a providers' perspective. Patient day equivalent (PDE) for tertiary and districts hospitals has been estimated elsewhere[18, 19], therefore findings of our study will add to this body of knowledge to determine PDE including palliative care for both tertiary and district hospitals in South Africa.

Methodology

Study Setting

Ethical approval for this study was obtained from the University of Cape Town Health Sciences' Human Research Ethics Committee (HREC REF 521/2019). The study was conducted in the Western Cape Province of South Africa, at Groote Schuur Hospital (GSH) a tertiary academic public hospital. GSH had an annual capacity of 43 031 inpatient admissions and 417 234 outpatients visits, with 893 beds in use (approximately 81% bed occupancy)[20]. There was an average of 525 doctors, 1 412 nurses and 268 allied health professionals employed to serve patients during the study period.

This study will only focus on the existing HBCPCS provided at GSH. The GSH palliative care team has been at the forefront in the development of the Western Cape palliative care policy which was launched in 2018. GSH including two other district hospitals are the only hospitals with operational hospital based palliative care services in the province, servicing eligible palliative care patients[21]. HBCPCS is not an admitting ward but a team consulting to all inpatient wards within the hospital. These services provide a comprehensive palliative care assessment, discharge planning, pain and symptom control with the treatment team together with psycho-social and spiritual support. The teams also liaise and refer to community-based services, for instance home-based care and hospices, to ensure continuity of care for palliative care patients: organise family meetings for education and counselling and provide bereavement counselling to families. Further, the team facilitates follow up phone calls and refers patients to social services including providing palliative care mentorship for health care workers within their respective facilities.

Data Collection

We collected costing data for 2019 using three data collection techniques: inventory audits, key informant interviews observations and inventory audits. We interviewed key informants who are involved in the delivery of palliative care services in GSH to understand comprehensively the services they offer, the times they work and collate key assets that were used in delivery of palliative care services. Inventory audits were used by researchers together with the palliative care team to identify and quantify recurrent and capital items. Capital items included durable medical equipment, furniture, and administrative equipment; and recurrent items: consumables, administrative stationery, all of which are used in production of the palliative care service in GSH. We identified, quantified and costed all inputs required in the production of HBCPCS including the cost of professional training for palliative care professionals (this is over and above their formal tertiary training such as their graduate and postgraduate degrees)[22]. We used a fulltime equivalent at 40 hours a week to account for the time spent by the fulltime clinical health and allied professionals that were directly linked to the HBCPCS delivery: key informant interviews were also used to determine other materials required for delivery of palliative care services from the providers perspective, such as training (treated as a capital item), conferences and in-kind contributions such as the kitchenware, family room and boardroom refurbishments. Observations were used by the researcher to follow the patients journey throughout the palliative care trajectory to identify inputs in the production of the service. All inputs required in the production of the HBCPCS were checked against the Gardiner et al. 2017 Framework (a systematic review which assessed data from many countries such as Canada, The United States of America and the United Kingdom among others)[22] to ensure that the cost estimates were as inclusive as possible. No personal data was included, such as salary data linked to specific persons, instead we estimated the salaries using the 2018/19 department public services and administration (DPSA) salary appendices according to job specifications and employment levels[23]. All identified assets were verified against the GSH main asset register compiled yearly by the asset department for management of assets. All costs are presented in 2019 South African Rands.

Data Analysis

We used a mixed method approach to estimate the unit cost of providing a HBCPCS in a tertiary hospital adopting a public provider perspective to determine an incremental cost associated with the provision of the HBCPCS (the additional amount required for HBCPCS provided over and above the hospitalization costs associated with the patient's admission). We developed a purpose-built costing tool in Microsoft Excel in consultation with palliative care specialists to estimate the cost of recurrent, capital and in-kind contributions in order to determine economic costs of delivering the HBCPCS in a tertiary public hospital. Recurrent items are those items with a life span of less than one year. While capital items are those items which have useful lives greater than one year. Capital items were annuitized using a rate of 3%[24]. We estimate in-kind labour costs by calculating the number of hours personnel worked over a defined period, and then using the standard market rate based on seniority and region we calculated the cost of their contribution to the production of the service. To determine the cost of different staff complements, we have performed a scenario analysis comparing the current practise at GSH to scenarios where the size of the team is scaled-up[25, 26]. For this study we only included patients that were assessed as eligible using the palliative care assessment tool, which in

2019 the total number of consultation or visits in the HBCPCS was 3985. This number denotes the denominator used for estimating the incremental unit cost. In the two broad categories of costs; recurrent and capital costs; researchers have identified ten categories of inputs for resources including a standard drug package *(see Table 1)*. We compared the costs (see Appendix 7, Supplementary Table, Table 2) with the findings of a study conducted by Hongoro et al. in 2011[17], which uses a similar methodology and was conducted in South Africa. Therefore, there was no need for using purchasing power parity to adjust costs. We used the South African consumer price index (CPI) to inflate the costs to the year presented[27].

Scenario Analysis

The palliative team in GSH is comprised of a medical doctor, a clinical nurse practitioner (CNP), a professional nurse (PN), two social auxiliary workers and administrative personnel. We performed a scenario analysis to estimate the cost of direct staff, if the staff complement was altered in the following ways: In Scenario A we added one CNP and two PNs to the existing staff. In Scenario B we added one GP, one CNP and one PN to the existing staff. While, in Scenario C we doubled the clinical staff number (i.e., two GPs, two CNPs, two PNs, four social auxiliary workers and one administrative personnel).

Results

In GSH there were 3 985 total palliative care encounters successfully conducted by the palliative care team between January and the end of December 2019. Of these 1 027 were inpatients registered and cared for by the palliative care team over the period, while 1 482 encounters were repeat consultations for patients that were already registered and who needed a follow-up consultation in the same episode of admission. A total of 50 patients were readmitted to the hospital and subsequently registered for a second palliative care consultation while hospitalized in the second episode of admission. The team facilitated 700 family meetings and 726 phone call encounters to follow-up with patients and to provide family support when patients were discharged making a total of 3985 encounters for the year 2019 *(see Figure 1 below)*.

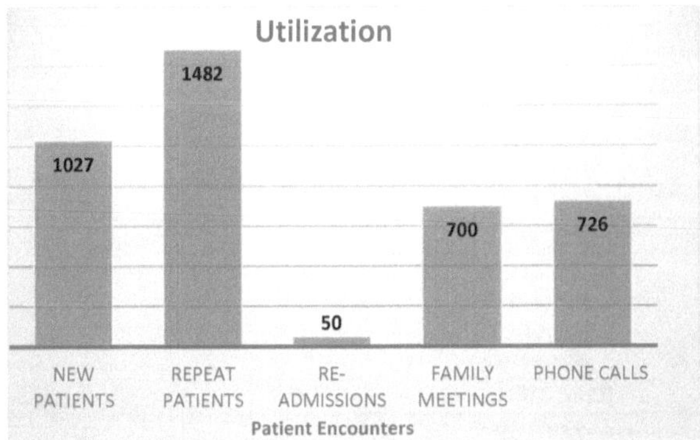

Figure 1: Utilization of HBCPCS in GSH

The total cost for running the HBCPCS was R2 494 419 accounting for both recurrent and capital costs. Recurrent items alone accounted for 96% (R2 392 407) of these costs (see Table 1). Personnel costs represented the greatest proportion of recurrent costs (91%) with direct personnel accounting for 89%, indirect and volunteering personnel accounting for 3% of the total cost. Running costs which included transportation, consumables and stationery accounted for a total of 4%. Capital items accounted for 4% (R102 013) during the study period, these including durable medical equipment (0.2%), furniture (1%), training of the team (2%) and non-labour in-kind contribution (0.5%). Capital costs had items with a life expectancy of between two and ten years (depending on the item) and were amortized at a 3% rate. The cost of the total medication list for palliative care was R3 185 (i.e., if one was to use one of each of the medications that are routinely prescribed), while a standard treatment package was R16 (per individual). The total cost per visit was found to be R626 without medication or R642 inclusive of the standard drug treatment package.

Table 1: Total annual cost by input

Recurrent	ZAR 2019	%
Personnel	**R2 281 887.74**	**91%**
Direct Staff	R2 213 079.00	89%
Indirect Staff	R68 808.74	3%
Other	**R110 518.90**	**4%**
Transportation	R67 650.00	3%
Consumables	R24 317.70	1%
Administration Stationary	R18 551.20	1%
Total Recurrent Cost	**R2 392 406.64**	**96%**
Capital	**ZAR 2019**	
Durable Medical Equipment	R4 443.30	0.2%
Furniture	R28 208.46	1%
Training	R58 024.05	2%
In-Kind Contributions Non-Labour	R11 336.64	0.5%
Total Capital Cost	**R102 012.45**	**4%**
Total Recurrent & Capital Cost	**R2 494 419.09**	

Scenario Analysis

The HBCPCS at GSH is team driven, direct staff constituted 89% of the total annual cost which represents R2.2 million. Direct staff are involved primarily in HBCPCS whereas indirect staff members are those who are in a supportive role to the palliative care team and constituted only 3% of the total annual cost. The results of the scenario analyses were as follows: Scenario A had a cost of R2.3 million; Scenario B had a cost close to R4 million; and Scenario C with double the number of the current palliative care staff would cost almost R4.4 million (*see Figure 2*).

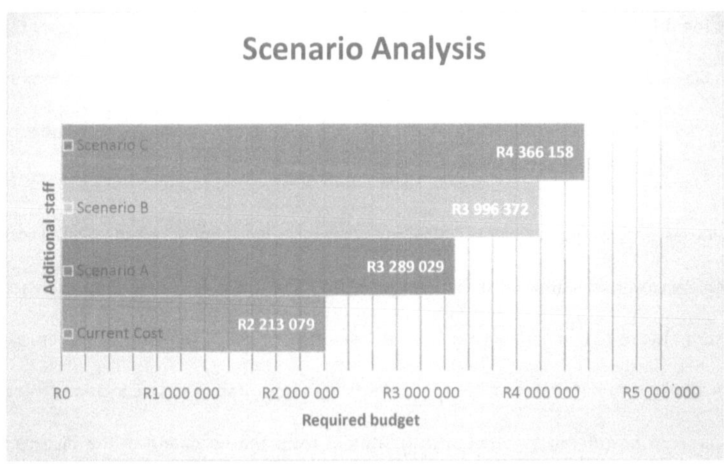

Figure 2: Scenario Analysis for staffing a HBCPCS.

Discussion

This study provides empirical evidence of the cost of consultative palliative care services in a tertiary public hospital in South Africa, the annual cost of this service being R2.4 million. We are unable to compare our incremental cost per visit (R642) to the cost of hospitalisation for an average patient day equivalent (PDE), as our cost is per visit regardless of the number of days that an inpatient receives HBCPCS. However for interest the PDE adjusted for the national mix of district, regional and tertiary hospital in 2011 was R2 237[(18)], inflated at a rate of 1.4 this represents R3 212 in 2019 South African Rands. For district hospitals the average patient day equivalent is R1 543[(19)] (inflated with a consumer price inflation rate of 1.4). This in contrast to the general medical ward in a private hospital of approximately R 3 768 (a minimum rate per day of R3 600[(28)] inflated using a consumer price inflation of rate 1.04). However, there are notable structural differences between public and private health care which can make huge cost disparity accounted for by purchasing and staffing arrangements so It is likely our estimated unit cost per visit for HBPCS would be an underestimation for the private sector. Adding per day palliative care services to these hospital inpatient costs would increase overall cost of the PDE however we theorise that this model of integration would be less than adding and running a comprehensive palliative care admitting ward or facility-based models. This finding is the first step in establishing whether efforts to establish lower-cost, affordable palliative care that is satisfactory for patients is possible in South Africa[29]. However, there is a need for a comprehensive economic evaluation in this field to investigate the cost effectiveness of palliative care strategies. Our findings, of a proportionally small incremental cost, are consistent with other costing studies HBCPCS seen in high income countries[30, 31], where palliative care services only has a small impact on the overall cost of hospitalization. However, research on palliative care shows that there is very limited evidence available for costing studies to compare with in Sub-Saharan Africa or LMICs generally[32]. It is crucial to have HBCPCS attached to hospitals that service patients with advanced disease conditions[33], so that palliative care can be offered together with treatment from the beginning of the disease's trajectory.

The findings of this study determined the costs of HBCPCS in a public hospital which is intended to provide decision makers with cost evidence which will hopefully allow for the prioritization of HBCPCS for inpatients in public hospitals. Interventions in health care are not chosen based on their costs or even cost-effectiveness alone, consideration about the value these services add on patients' lives is also necessary. Improved palliative care coverage should provide palliative care wherever patients are homes, communities and in hospitals. It is important to have these services for outpatients and home-based patients, so that the needs of these patients are catered closer to where they reside. When dealing with a diverse population such as in South Africa, there is no one model that fits all individuals, especially when considering rolling out a comprehensive palliative care policy in a country with wider economic disparities. However, palliative care models should be evaluated for both cost and effectiveness where possible[34], in order to provide decision-makers with the necessary evidence to determine which strategies have the best outcomes and which the country can best afford. We cannot overlook palliative care in South Africa, considering both the burden of diseases, the financial loss palliative care place on individuals or household and for other reasons stated elsewhere[35-37].

Hospital based palliative care service are less costly than hospital-based outreach services. However, they are only accessible to a relatively small subset of the population[30, 38]. The GSH HBCPCS supports palliative care eligible patients who are admitted in this tertiary hospital, the team also supports families with the necessary tools when the patients are discharged and provides bereavement counselling when needed which are all invaluable and essential services. The HBCPCS is not an admitting ward but rather a team of health and allied health professionals consulting to various wards within the hospital, and for this reason we have observed that personnel was a major cost driver for this service accounting for 91% of the total running costs. This study established an incremental costing of the HBCPCS at GSH, where we deliberately excluded infrastructure (mainly building costs) and overheads (such as water, electricity, and maintenance etc.) to establish a cost for running HBCPCS over and above the hospitalization costs. The total cost of running the service at GSH was R2.4 million accounting for only 0.005% of the total national healthcare spending for the 2019/20 fiscal year[29-31, 39].

The HBCPCS was less costly when compared to a similar strategy (HBOPCS) provided in Chris Baragwanath hospital in the Gauteng Province. The HBOPCS has an annual running cost of R11 million[17], while, the findings of our study suggest that HBCPCS can delivered in a tertiary hospital with a cost of R2.4 million. Hongoro and Dinat's (2011) cost analysis accounted for recurrent items only, which makes it comparable to our findings given that we have used an incremental costing technique. The differences in costs between these two studies (Hongoro et al. (2011) and ours) can be attributed to many reasons: HBCPCS at GSH does not require intensive medical equipment; provides service to inpatients only; and the only major input in HBCPCS was personnel but even so the staff complement was smaller than the HBOPCS. The team in GSH was composed of one doctor, one clinical nurse practitioner, one professional nurse, two social auxiliary workers and one admin personnel. The composition of the team was working at full capacity, which contributed to the available staff being overworked and sometimes some of the key functions of the services not being given the time and dedication they warrant such as education, research and training of other professionals within the hospital. The research component especially for economic evaluation of palliative care interventions has not been focused on in LMICs, as evidenced by the lack of published studies in the field in many African countries[32]. While published research shows that there has been many attempts in establishing costing frameworks and in conducting cost-effectiveness and cost analysis for palliative care interventions in high income countries[39].

As a larger team may be necessary to perform HBCPCS we conducted scenario analyses of several scaled-up options. As expected, when individuals higher in the organogram of HBCPCS are added to the team, the overall budgetary need is increased. These scenarios are based on ideal expert opinions. However, further studies are required to determine the best alternatives for staffing complement in the delivery of palliative care services. Calculating staffing requirements for specialized palliative care services is an intricate task and there is little literature published to suggest best practice. However, according to Henderson et al. (2019), staffing hospital that provides palliative care depends largely on the number of patient referrals and on expert opinion. They recommend at least one full time equivalent (FTE) registered nurse, one FTE physician and 0.5 FTE social worker for every 25 referrals in a single month[40]. While, the Western Cape Policy and Strategy on Palliative Care proposes one dedicated palliative care specialist (academic posts), one or two dedicated doctors (medical officer level), five dedicated palliative care nurses, two social workers, five axillary social workers and an administrator[41]. We are providing this cost information with the intension that decision makers will better understand the cost drivers, resources required and affordability of palliative care interventions amidst the scarce resources in healthcare to innovate as it has been done elsewhere [35].

Additional to direct staff there were other personnel who were not directly involved in the palliative care services such as occupational therapists, physiotherapists, dieticians, speech therapist, social workers, among others. Once the palliative care team carries out the palliative care assessment these personnel were often consulted occasionally to offer additional services to patients with palliative care needs. These staff are integral to the care given and only represent a small percentage of the overall cost (indirect staff accounted only for 3% of the total cost of the service).

Furthermore, the palliative care team is given ad hoc training in palliative care to refresh and improve their knowledge. The auxiliary workers in the HBCPCS have been trained together with other personnel in palliative care to improve their competencies. This is a team of champions who provide mentorship to other institutions in the district, but if the team considers scaling up it would better to consider social workers instead since they would be on a same competency level and this would avoid training costs for auxiliary workers. It was necessary for this study to reflect the cost of training for professional staff understanding the value training has added to the quality of the services, it is through these investments that we see improved quality in services provision. Training has a critical significance in developing an adequately skilled workforce, training however accounted for only a small proportion of the total cost of the service (2%).

The team also facilitated family meetings and performed follow-up phone calls to reintegrate the patients with their family while also ensuring that the family was able to provide the necessary support to be able to take care of their loved ones and felt supported themselves. Furthermore, recommendations and placements of patients to hospices was facilitated by the palliative care team in instances where the patients were not managed at home following their hospital discharge [21] . In 2019 alone there were 58 patients that were placed in hospices, based on this number cost of transportation of these patients was 3% of the total cost of this service.

Limited medical equipment was required for HBCPCS hence the proportion of the cost is low. In many medical interventions personnel and medical equipment are the major drivers for many services. However, in this service we have observed only personnel being the major cost driver as the medical and surgical wards are the holders of the larger medical equipment in the hospital and therefore a responsibility of the admitting ward since the palliative care team is consultatory. We formulated a standard prescription and costed this package separately so that it could be added subsequently to the unit cost of a HBCPCS visit, and easily changed if the medication or cost of medication changed dramatically. There was no treatment administered to patients directly by the team, instead the palliative care doctor writes a prescription which is given at the pharmacy based on availability. There is no substitute for HBCPCS within hospitals, the value they add to the patient's quality of life is unmatched, and we have shown the monetary cost of this to be low. The GSH palliative care team has been an example to other institutions and in the forefront of the palliative care policy launch in the Western Cape.

Conclusion

HBCPCS are essential especially when linked to surgical, medical, oncology and other intensive care inpatient wards. These services may be provided alongside treatment to patients with chronic disease conditions to improve quality of life of these patients at the end of life. The role of the palliative care team extends beyond clinical care to further connecting these patients to ward based outreach teams and placing these patients in hospices. With an aging population and the observed disease burden in South Africa it is impossible to overlook palliative care. Our findings shows that HBCPCS can be offered with just R2.4 million in one tertiary public hospital over a year, and with this cost these services can be offered simultaneously with other modalities of palliative care to provide a comprehensive approach of palliative care and to cater for patients in hospitals. This study provides the cost component of HBCPCS, paving a way for further research specifically cost analyses of palliative care interventions at different levels of care, as understanding the cost component can provide an opportunity for innovation in resource allocation. Adding on to this body of work we recommend a rigorous cost-effectiveness analysis for these interventions in low- and middle-income countries in order to better the value the options.

Declaration

The authors have no conflict of interests to declare.

References

1. Rhee JY, Garralda E, Namisango E, Luyirika E, de Lima L, Powell RA, et al. Factors Affecting Palliative Care Development in Africa: In-Country Experts' Perceptions in Seven Countries. Journal of pain and symptom management. 2018;55(5):1313-20.e2.
2. Rhee JY, Garralda E, Torrado C, Blanco S, Ayala I, Namisango E, et al. Palliative care in Africa: a scoping review from 2005-16. The Lancet Oncology. 2017;18(9):e522-e31.
3. Sasaki H, Bouesseau M-C, Marston J, Mori R. A scoping review of palliative care for children in low-and middle-income countries. BMC palliative care. 2017;16(1):60.
4. Frankenfeld P. One year mortality after hospital admission as an indicator of palliative care need in the Western Cape, South Africa: an incident cohort study [Quantitative Study]: University of Cape Town 2020.
5. WHA67 R. 19. Strengthening of palliative care as a component of comprehensive care throughout the life course. 2014.
6. NDoH. National Policy Framework and Stratergy on Palliative Care 2017-2022. In: DoH, editor. Pretoria: National Department of Health; 2017.
7. Msemburi W, Pillay-van Wyk V, Dorrington R, E, Neethling I, Nannan N, Groenewald P, et al. Second national burden of disease study for South Africa: Cause-of-death profile for South Africa, 1997–2010.; 2014. Report No.: 978-1-920618-34-6.
8. Pillay-van Wyk V, Msemburi W, Laubscher R, Dorrington RE, Groenewald P, Glass T, et al. Mortality trends and differentials in South Africa from 1997 to 2012: second National Burden of Disease Study. The Lancet Global Health. 2016;4(9):e642-e53.
9. Ali Z. Integrating Palliative Care in Cancer Care in Kenya. Journal of Global Oncology. 2018;4(Supplement 2):164s-s.
10. Nanney E, Smith S, Hartwig K, Mmbando P. Scaling up palliative care services in rural Tanzania. Journal of pain and symptom management. 2010;40(1):15-8.
11. Mortality Database on data reported to WHO as of 31 December 2019 [Internet]. WHO. 2019. Available from: https://app.powerbi.com/view?r=eyJrIjoiZjYzN2Q0YjgtYTlhYi00NjQwLTliMWMtZWM0ZGI4OWQwN2YzIiwidCI6ImNkNmU2NTQ5LWMwZGYtNDc4Ny04OWVjLTVmYTk0OGI2YTIzZCIsImMiOjh9.
12. van Niekerk L, Raubenheimer PJ. A point-prevalence survey of public hospital inpatients with palliative care needs in Cape Town, South Africa. S Afr Med J. 2014;104(2):138-41.
13. Connor SR. Global Atlas of Pallitiave Care. World Health Organization; 2020.
14. Frankenfeld P NvL, Manning K, Tiffin N, Raubenheimer P.J. One year mortality after hospital admission as an indicator of palliative care need in South Africa: incident cohort study 2019.
15. Sepúlveda C, Marlin A, Yoshida T, Ullrich A. Palliative Care: the World Health Organization's global perspective. J Pain Symptom Manage. 2002;24(2):91-6.
16. Vassall A, Sweeney S, Kahn J, Gomez Guillen G, Bollinger L, Marseille E, et al. Reference case for estimating the costs of global health services and interventions. 2017.
17. Hongoro C, Dinat N. A cost analysis of a hospital-based palliative care outreach program: implications for expanding public sector palliative care in South Africa. J Pain Symptom Manage. 2011;41(6):1015-24.
18. Ramjee S. Comparing the Cost of Delivering Hospital Services across the Public and Private Sectors in South Africa. The Hospital Association of South Africa, University of Cape Town. 2013.
19. Day C, Budgell E, Gray A. Health and related indicators. South African health review. 2011;2011(1):119-248.
20. Goverment WC. Fast Facts GSH. In: health Do, editor. Cape Town 2009.
21. Gwyther L, Krause R, Cupido C, Stanford J, Grey H, Credé T, et al. The development of hospital-based palliative care services in public hospitals in the Western Cape, South Africa. South African Medical Journal. 2018;108(2):86-9.

22. Gardiner C, Ingleton C, Ryan T, Ward S, Gott M. What cost components are relevant for economic evaluations of palliative care, and what approaches are used to measure these costs? A systematic review. Palliative medicine. 2017;31(4):323-37.
23. DPSA. Appendix B to Department Public Service and Adminitration Circular 10 of 2018. In: Administration DPSa, editor. 2018.
24. Netten A, Knight J. Annuitizing the human capital investment costs of health service professionals. Health Economics. 1999;8(3):245-55.
25. Henderson JD, Boyle A, Herx L, Alexiadis A, Barwich D, Connidis S, et al. Staffing a Specialist Palliative Care Service, a Team-Based Approach: Expert Consensus White Paper. Journal of palliative medicine. 2019;22(11):1318-23.
26. WHO. Planning and implementing palliative care services: a guide for programme managers. 2016.
27. StatsSA. CPI headline year-on-year rates. In: CPIHistory.pdf, editor. South Africa: STATISTICS SA; 2016.
28. Holding L. Cost of a bed in private hospitals in 2018. In: Mbuthini L, editor. Email ed2019.
29. Reid EA, Kovalerchik O, Jubanyik K, Brown S, Hersey D, Grant L. Is palliative care cost-effective in low-income and middle-income countries? A mixed-methods systematic review. BMJ supportive & palliative care. 2019;9(2):120-9.
30. Smith S, Brick A, O'Hara S, Normand C. Evidence on the cost and cost-effectiveness of palliative care: a literature review. Palliative medicine. 2014;28(2):130-50.
31. Penrod JD, Deb P, Dellenbaugh C, Burgess Jr JF, Zhu CW, Christiansen CL, et al. Hospital-based palliative care consultation: effects on hospital cost. Journal of palliative medicine. 2010;13(8):973-9.
32. Pastrana T, Vallath N, Mastrojohn J, Namukwaya E, Kumar S, Radbruch L, et al. Disparities in the contribution of low-and middle-income countries to palliative care research. Journal of pain and symptom management. 2010;39(1):54-68.
33. Hannon B, Zimmermann C, Knaul FM, Powell RA, Mwangi-Powell FN, Rodin G. Provision of palliative care in low-and middle-income countries: overcoming obstacles for effective treatment delivery. J Clin Oncol. 2016;34(1):62-8.
34. Bickel K, Ozanne E. Importance of Costs and Cost Effectiveness of Palliative Care. Journal of oncology practice. 2017;13(5):287.
35. Anderson RE, Grant L. What is the value of palliative care provision in low-resource settings? BMJ global health. 2017;2(1).
36. Coleman AM. Palliative Care, Suffering, Death Trajectory: A View of End-of-Life Care (EOL) Related Issues in Sub-Saharan Africa (SSA). International Journal of Clinical Medicine. 2018;9(3):175-81.
37. Bates MJ, Namisango E, Tomeny E, Muula A, Squire SB, Niessen L. Palliative care within universal health coverage: the Malawi Patient-and-Carer Cancer Cost Survey. BMJ supportive & palliative care. 2019:bmjspcare-2019-001945.
38. Africa SS. CPI: headline index numbers.
39. Smith S, Brick A, O'Hara S, Normand C. Evidence on the cost and cost-effectiveness of palliative care: a literature review. Palliative medicine. 2014;28(2):130-50.
40. Staffing a Specialist Palliative Care Service, a Team-Based Approach: Expert Consensus White Paper. Journal of palliative medicine. 2019;22(11):1318-23.
41. DoH W. proposed model for the implementation of palliative care policy in the Western Cape In: DoH W, editor. 2018.

PART D: POLICY BRIEF

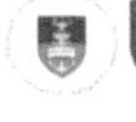
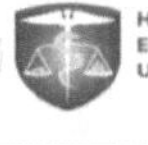

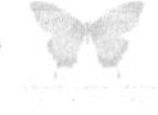

Policy Brief 2020

The cost of providing consultative palliative care services in a tertiary public hospital setting in South Africa

This policy brief reports the cost of providing a hospital based consultative palliative care service (HBCPCS) for a tertiary public hospital in South Africa.

Key Findings

- ✓ The palliative care team in Groote Schuur Hospital is composed of; one doctor, one clinical nurse practitioner, one professional nurse, two social auxiliary workers and one administrative personnel.
- ✓ The role of palliative care team extends beyond clinical care to further connecting and placing patients to outreach teams and hospices following their hospital discharge.
- ✓ There were 3 985 total patient consultations between January-December 2019. The total cost of this service was R2.4 million. Whilst, a cost per visit was R642 including a standard drug package(1).
- ✓ The total cost of running the HBCPCS accounted for only 0.005% of the total national healthcare spending for the 2019/20 fiscal year

Introduction

Given the burden of disease in South Africa and the World Health Organization (WHO) recommendation to integrate palliative care services we cannot overlook palliative care services. The Sub-Saharan region has sparse established palliative care to cater to people with complex symptoms due to life-limiting conditions or terminal illnesses. Palliative care aims to enhance and preserve quality of life for patients and their loved ones and encourages them to live as actively as possible while they are alive.

The top mortality trends in the Western Cape Province (WC) resonate with the burden of disease profile in South Africa generally(2). Considering the window of opportunity presented by the introduction of universal health coverage and the burden of disease faced in the region, it is now an opportune moment to grant palliative care the recognition it deserves. These statistics show a great need for palliative care interventions for the general population and especially for those patients who suffer from life limiting-illnesses.

Methodology

The study was conducted in the WC, at Groote Schuur Hospital (GSH) a teaching tertiary-level public hospital. We have used a mixed method to estimate the incremental unit cost of providing HBCPCS adopting a public provider's perspective. We costed recurrent and capital items used in the production of the HBCPCS, a combination of assets inventory, key informant interviews and observations were used to collect this empirical costing data. These costs were captured for the 2018/19 fiscal year and included the annual operational cost and cost per visit for the service. The cost of capital items (with a life expectancy exceeding one year) were annuitized using a 3% rate and combined with recurrent cost to establish the incremental cost of HBCPCS (above the cost of hospitalization).

Findings

The major cost driver in the HBCPCS was direct personnel which accounted for 91% of the total cost. This finding mirrored what was happening on the ground, the service is not an admitting ward but rather a team of health professionals consulting in various wards within the hospital. When we performed a scenario analysis for scaling-up options, we have observed that doubling the number of the clinical and allied staff would increase the cost to R4.4 million. The findings of this study shows that one HBCPCS accounted for 0.005% of the total national healthcare spending for the 2019/20 fiscal year.

This policy brief was prepared: Mr. Linda. Mbuthini **Supervised by**: Ms. Lucy Cunnama, Dr René Krause and Prof Jennifer Moodley

Table 1: Total annual cost by input

Recurrent	ZAR 2019	%
Personnel	**R2 281 887.74**	91%
Direct Staff	R2 213 079.00	89%
Indirect Staff	R68 808.74	3%
Other	**R110 518.90**	4%
Transportation	R67 650.00	3%
Consumables	R24 317.70	1%
Administration Stationary	R18 551.20	1%
Total Recurrent Cost	**R2 392 406.64**	**96%**
Capital	**ZAR 2019**	
Durable Medical Equipment	R4 443.30	0.2%
Furniture	R28 208.46	1%
Training	R58 024.05	2%
In-kind Contributions Non-labour	R11 336.64	0.5%
Total Capital Cost	**R102 012.45**	**4%**
Total Recurrent & Capital Cost	**R2 494 419.09**	

When we compared this service (HBCPCS) to a hospital based outreach palliative care services (HBOPCS)[3], we observed that HBCPCS is less expensive. HBCPCS are essential especially when linked to; surgical, medical, oncology and other intensive care inpatient wards. While, these inpatient services improve health, palliative care improves dignity and quality of life for patients facing life-limiting conditions, and their families. There were notable vacancies in the structure of the team, which contributed to the available staff being overworked and sometimes some of the key functions of the services being overlooked such as research into palliative care and training of other staff. Furthermore, this team provides mentorship to other institutions in the province and they have played a vital role in the development of the proposed model for the implementation of palliative care policy in the WC. The role of the palliative care team extends beyond clinical care to further connecting these patients to ward based outreach teams and placing these patients in hospices for continuity of care, the team also supports families; teaches them how to care for their loved ones; and provides bereavement counselling. These finding show that HBCPCS are potentially of low cost when run in a public tertiary hospital and may be of huge benefit to patients and their families.

Recommendations

HBCPCS can be offered simultaneously with other modalities of palliative care to provide a comprehensive approach which caters to patients with life-limiting conditions or terminal illnesses. It is crucial to provide HBCPCS in hospitals that service patients with advanced disease conditions, so that palliative care can be offered together with treatment from the beginning of the disease's trajectory. Given the low proportion of the HBCPCS to the national healthcare expenditure, this modality can be provided in other tertiary facilities within the country.

References

1. Mbuthini L, Cunnama L, Krause R, Moodley J. The cost of providing consultative palliative care services in a tertiary hospital setting: The case of Groote Schuur Hospital. 2020.
2. van Niekerk L, Raubenheimer PJ. A point-prevalence survey of public hospital inpatients with palliative care needs in Cape Town, South Africa. S Afr Med J. 2014;104(2):138-41.
3. Hongoro C, Dinat N. A cost analysis of a hospital-based palliative care outreach program: implications for expanding public sector palliative care in South Africa. J Pain Symptom Manage. 2011;41(6):1015-24.

This policy brief was prepared: Mr. Linda. Mbuthini **Supervised by**: Ms. Lucy Cunnama, Dr René Krause and Prof Jennifer Moodley

PART E: APPENDICES

Appendix 1: Study Budget

Costing HBPCS GSH
Period: 06 Months
Partner: University of Cape Town (HEU), GSH Palliative Care Unit & Western Cape DoH

	Rate/Hour	Description of unit cost	Quantities	Description of quantity	Frequency	Description of frequency	
Item	**Base Cost (ZAR)**	**Comment**	**Qty**	**Comment**	**Frequency**	**Comment**	**Total (ZAR)**
Personnel							
Data Collector	R 85	per hour	40	Hour p/m	1	months	R 3 400
Editor	R 120	per hour	10	Hour p/m	2	months	R 2 400
Subtotal: Personnel							**R 5 800**
Research costs							
Material	R 1 500						
Printing	R 400						
Subtotal: Research costs	**R 1 900**						
Equipment							
1 x Laptops	R 10 000						
1 x Back packs	R 300						
Subtotal: Equipment	**R 10 300**						
Supplies							
Stationery	R 500						
Subtotal: Supplies	**R 500**						
Travel							
Flights	R -	per flight	0	people	0	trips	R -
Accommodation	R -	per person pe	0	people x days	0	trips	R -
Per diem	R -	per person pe	0	people x days	0	trips	R -
Vehicle hire	R -	daily rate	0	days	0	trips	R -
Transport cost for data collection	R 150	per transfer	1	people x days	3	trips	R 450
Conference registration		per trip	1	car	1	trips	R -
Subtotal: Travel							**R 450**
Training & capacity building							
	R -						
Subtotal: Training	**R -**						
Other							
Data & Airtime	R 200						
Subtotal: Other	**R 200**						
Indirect Costs							
Indirect costs	R 19 150	total budget	20%	percentage	1	per year	R 3 830
Subtotal: Indirect costs							**R 3 830**
Total: All Categories							**R 22 980**

Appendix 2: Study Timelines

Stages	Activities	Year	2019						2020					
		Month	Jan-Feb	Mar-April	May-June	Jul-Aug	Sep- Oct	Nov-Dec	Jan-Feb	Mar-April	May-June	Jul-Aug	Sep- Oct	Nov-Dec
Phase 1	Study Protocol and Work Plan Development													
	Ethics submission and approval													
	Development of Costing tool & Validation													
Phase 2	Data Collection													
	Data validation													
Phase 3	Data Analyses													
	Write-up													
Pase 4	Submission for publication													
	Conference attendance													
	Closure													

Appendix 3: Palliative Care Assessment Form

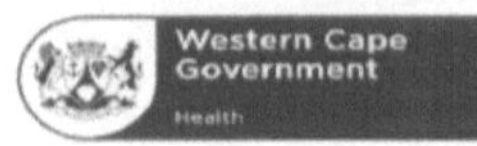

Adult Form

Palliative Care Assessment

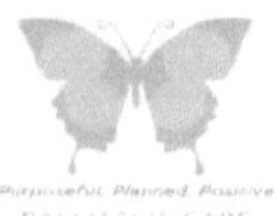

Admission date:	Discharge date:
PC referral date:	Re-admission date:
PC assessment date:	Date of death:
Referring ward	Place of death:
Consent to be part of database? ☐ yes ☐ no	☐ unable Reason:
Referring doctor:	Responsible pc member:
Doctor's mobile no.:	PC member's mobile no.:
Doctor's email:	PC member's email:
PATIENT INFORMATION (place sticker or complete information)	
Folder number:	Date of birth:
Surname:	Contact number:
First name:	Home language: Gender:
Address:	
NEXT OF KIN INFORMATION (please complete as detailed as possible)	
Folder number:	Relation to patient
Contact no 1:	Contact no 2:
Physical address:	

Referral location:

☐ Surgery ☐ OB/Gynae ☐ Orthopaedics ☐ Trauma ☐ ICU ☐ ED
☐ Medical ☐ Renal clinic ☐ Medical Outpatient ☐ Surgery outpatient ☐ Oncology ☐ Other

Reasons for referral:

☐ Pain management ☐ Other symptom management ☐ Home base care ☐ Syringe driver ☐ BBN
☐ Transfer to other facility ☐ Counselling for patient/family ☐ Education ☐ Hospice referral/discussion
☐ Other:

Primary diagnoses:

☐ Cancer (solid tumour) ______________ ☐ Vascular ☐ Infectious/TB/HIV ☐ Haematology ☐ Frailty
☐ Neurologic/stroke ☐ Hepatic ☐ Cardiovascular ☐ Trauma
☐ Progressive neurological conditions ☐ Pulmonary ☐ Renal ☐ Dementia
☐ Other:

History:

ECOG performance status: ☐ 1(mobile) ☐ 2 ☐ 3 ☐ Fully Bedbound

Mental status: ☐ Orientated ☐ Confused ☐ Unconscious ☐ Fluctuating GCS

Patient understanding diagnosis ☐ yes ☐ no Understanding prognosis ☐ yes ☐ no

Family informed ☐ yes ☐ no

Symptom/Needs Assessment

Needs / Symptoms	Not screened	Negative	Positive	Grade (Scale)	Action Taken
Pain					
Non-pain symptoms					
Psychological needs					
Social					
Economic					
Spiritual					
Family support					

Scale Key: None: 0 Mild: 1 Moderate: 2 Severe: 3 Not assessed: 7 Unable to rate: 9

PC Team's Contact Person:

PC Team's Contact number: Contact email:

Appendix 4: Written informed consent for Key Informant Interviews

The cost of providing consultative palliative care services in a tertiary hospital setting

This study is conducted by Linda Mbuthini from the University of Cape Town, Health Economics Unit, School of public health and family medicine, for a master's book with the possibility to publish results in the future.

The purpose of the study is to determine the costs and cost drivers for hospital based consultative palliative care service (HBPCS) in South Africa adopting a providers' perspective. Once the cost evidence has been established it may be used by decision makers to advocate for the integration of palliative care services in the general health care services.

Key informants who work in palliative care unit at Grote Schuur Hospital who give informed consent will take part in the study in order to give information regarding working times, general services and patients' palliative care needs. Questions will be asked, and the answers will be recorded in the Microsoft excel spreadsheet tool. The interviews will take approximately 1 hour. There will be no follow up interview.

Participants may withdraw from the study at any stage. Feedback of results will be available to participants on request. There will be no risks, benefits nor cost involved for the participants in this study. There is no insurance cover for participants in this study as there are no anticipated harm.

Ethical approval for this study has been secured from The Faculty of Health Sciences Human Research Ethics Committee. All the research will adhere to the Declaration of Helsinki 2008. Participants can contact the Human Research Ethics Committee if there are any questions about their rights and welfare as research subjects.

If there are any further questions with regards to the study feel free to contact Linda Mbuthini MBTLIN006@myUCT.ac.a or cell number 0833100391.

I ____________________________have read the information sheet

(or it has been read to me by ______________________).

I understand what is required of me and I have had all my questions answered. I do not feel that I am forced to take part in this study and I am doing so of my own free will. I know that I can withdraw at any time if I so wish without any repercussions.

Signed: ____

Participant: _________________________ Date and place: __________________
Researcher: _________________________ Date and place: __________________
Witness: _________________________ Date and place: __________________

Appendix 5: Human Research Ethics Approval Letter

UNIVERSITY OF CAPE TOWN
Faculty of Health Sciences
Human Research Ethics Committee

Room E53-46 Old Main Buildin
Groote Schuur Hospit:
Observatory 792
Telephone [021] 406 649
Email: sumayah.ariefdien@uct.ac.z
Website: www.health.uct.ac.za/fhs/research/humanethics/form

26 August 2019

HREC REF: 521/2019

Ms L Cunnama
Division of Health Economics Unit
School of Public Health & Family Medicine
FHS

Dear Ms Cunnama

PROJECT TITLE: THE COST OF PROVIDING CONSULTATIVE PALLIATIVE CARE SERVICES IN A TERTIARY HOSPITAL SETTING: THE CASE OF GROOTE SCHUUR HOSPITAL (MASTERS CANDIDATE - MR L MBUTHINI)

Thank you for submitting your study to the Faculty of Health Sciences Human Research Ethics Committee (HREC) for review.

It is a pleasure to inform you that the HREC has **formally approved** the above-mentioned study.

Approval is granted for one year until the 30 August 2020.

Please submit a progress form, using the standardised Annual Report Form if the study continues beyond the approval period. Please submit a Standard Closure form if the study is completed within the approval period.
(Forms can be found on our website: www.health.uct.ac.za/fhs/research/humanethics/forms)

We acknowledge that the student: Mr Linda Mbuthini will also be involved in this study.

Please quote the HREC REF in all your correspondence.

Please note that the ongoing ethical conduct of the study remains the responsibility of the principal investigator.

Please note that for all studies approved by the HREC, the principal investigator **must** obtain appropriate institutional approval, where necessary, before the research may occur.

Yours sincerely

Signature Removed

PROFESSOR M BLOCKMAN
CHAIRPERSON, FHS HUMAN RESEARCH ETHICS COMMITTEE

Federal Wide Assurance Number: FWA00001637.
Institutional Review Board (IRB) number: IRB00001938

NHREC-registration number: REC-210208-007

This serves to confirm that the University of Cape Town Human Research Ethics Committee complies to the Ethics Standards for Clinical Research with a new drug in patients, based on the Medical Research Council (MRC-SA), Food and Drug Administration (FDA-USA), International Council for Harmonisation of Technical Requirements for Pharmaceuticals for Human Use: Good Clinical Practice (ICH GCP), South African Good Clinical Practice Guidelines (DoH 2006), based on the Association of the British Pharmaceutical Industry Guidelines (ABPI), and Declaration of Helsinki (2013) guidelines. The Human Research Ethics Committee granting this approval is in compliance with the ICH Harmonised Tripartite Guidelines E6: Note for Guidance on Good Clinical Practice (CPMP/ICH/135/95) and FDA Code Federal Regulation Part 50, 56 and 312.

Appendix 6: Department of Health Approval Letter

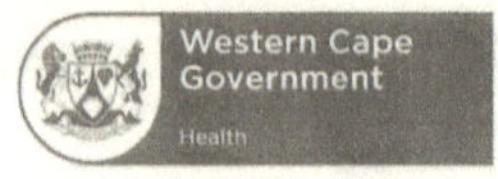

GROOTE SCHUUR HOSPITAL
Enquiries: Dr Bernadette Eick
e-mail: Bernadette.Eick@westerncape.gov.za

Ms. Lucy Cunnama
DIVISION OF HEALTH ECONOMICS – PUBLIC HEALTH & FAMILY MEDICINE

E-mail: Lucy.Cunnama@uct.ac.z.a / Linda.Mbuthini@uct.ac.za / Rene.Krause@uct.ac.za

Dear Ms. Cunnama,

RESEARCH PROJECT: The Cost of Providing Consultative palliative Care services in a tertiary hospital setting: The case of Groote Schuur Hospital (Masters Candidate Mr Linda Mbuthini)

Your recent letter to the hospital refers.

You are granted permission to proceed with your research, which is valid until **30 August 2020.**

Please note the following:

a) Your research may not interfere with normal patient care.
b) Hospital staff may not be asked to assist with the research.
c) No additional costs to the hospital should be incurred i.e. Lab, consumables or stationary. **If access to TRACK Care/NHLS is required, kindly attach our letter of approval to the application form.**
d) **No patient folders may be removed from the premises or be inaccessible.**
e) Please provide the research assistant/field worker with a copy of this letter as verification of approval.
f) Confidentiality must always be maintained .
g) Should you at any time require photographs of your subjects, please obtain the necessary indemnity forms from our Public Relations Office (E45 OMB or ext. 2187/2188).
h) Should you require additional research time beyond the stipulated expiry date, please apply for an extension.
i) Please discuss the study with the HOD before commencing.
j) Please introduce yourself to the person in charge of an area before commencing.
k) On completion of your research, please forward any recommendations/findings that can be beneficial to use to take further action that may inform redevelopment of future policy / review guidelines.
l) Kindly submit a copy of the publication or report to this office on completion of the research.
m) At no time should any posters encouraging patients to partake in research, be displayed within a clinical area.

I would like to wish you every success with the project.

Yours sincerely

Signature Removed

DR BERNADETTE EICK
CHIEF OPERATIONAL OFFICER
Date: 25 September 2019

C.C. Mr. L. Naidoo
Dr L. Booyens
Professor P. Raubenheimer

G46 Management Suite, Old Main Building,
Observatory 7925
Tel: +27 21 404 6288 fax: +27 21 404 6125

Private Bag X,
Observatory, 7935
www.westerncape.gov.za/health

Appendix 7: Supplementary Table

Table 2: Supplementary table- Total Recurrent Costs by Line Item (2019) HBCPCS vs HBPCOP

HBCPCS Groote Schuur		
Recurrent Items	**ZAR 2019**	**%**
Direct Staff	R2 213 079.00	93%
Indirect Staff	R68 808.74	3%
Transportation	R67 650.00	3%
Consumables	R24 317.70	1%
Administration Stationary	R18 551.20	1%
Total	**R2 392 406.64**	

HBPCOP Chris Baragwanath Hongoro et.al 2011		
Recurrent Items	**USD 2007**	**%**
Personnel	$441 991.50	63%
Costs and expenses	$102 455.31	15%
Project costs	$87 373.97	12%
Management support services	$70 201.09	10%
Total	**$702 021.87**	
Total HBPCOP **ZAR 2019***	**R11 063 864.67**	

Cost per visit		
	Total Encounters	**Cost Per visit**
HBCPCS	3985	R600.35
HBPCOP	7905	R1 399.60
Total Cost using standard number of encounters		
HBCPCS	5945	R402.42
HBPCOP	5945	R1 861.04

***(CPI 2019/CPI 2007)= (112/57)=1.97;**

Currency exchange in 2007 1 USD is equal 8 ZAR =$702 021.87*8 =R5 616 174.96;

1.97 * R5 616 174.96= R11 063 864.67

Appendix 8: Instructions for Authors

Guide and Instruction for Authors

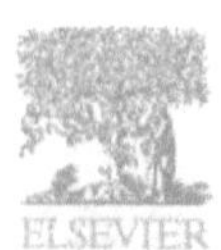

JOURNAL OF PAIN AND SYMPTOM MANAGEMENT
Advancing Palliative Care, Hospice, and Symptom Research

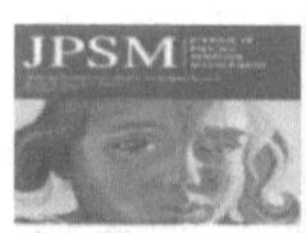

ISSN: 0885-3924

The Journal of Pain and Symptom Management is an internationally respected, peer-reviewed j serves an interdisciplinary audience of professionals by providing a forum for the publication of the latest clinical research and best practices related to the **relief** of **illness burden** among patients afflicted with **serious** or **life-threatening illness**.

The Journal has strongly supported both quantitative and qualitative research underpinning the evolving discipline of **palliative care**, including clinical trials of pain or **symptom control therapies**, epidemiology of phenomena related to life-threatening disease and **end-of-life care**, instrument development to enhance clinical assessment and facilitate investigation, and **health services** studies evaluating the outcomes of diverse **therapeutic models.** It also offers extensive coverage of clinical practice issues, publishing both systematic and narrative reviews, case series and case reports, and both special articles and columns that present important updates on topics as varied as the international diversity of **palliative medicine**, the economics of palliative care, and bioethics in end-of-life care.

AUDIENCE

Clinicians and Researchers working in pain management, palliative care or hospice care, including Oncologists, Anesthesiologists, Neurologists, Pharmacologists, Nurses, Therapists, Psychologists, and Psychiatrists.

IMPACT FACTOR

2018: 3.378 © Clarivate Analytics Journal Citation Reports 2019

ABSTRACTING AND INDEXING

Pub
Me
d/
Me
dlin
e
Em
bas
e
Psy
cIN
FO

Child Development Abstracts and
Bibliography Nursing Abstracts

International Nursing
Index Elsevier BIOBASE

Oncology Information Service

Cumulative Index to Nursing and Allied Health Literature
Current Contents - Clinical Medicine

Research Alert

Psych INFO, SciSearch,
MEDLARS Scopus

GUIDE FOR AUTHORS

Types of Articles

The *Journal of Pain and Symptom Management* publishes the following types of articles:

Note: JPSM publishes descriptions of original research findings in multiple sections. Please submit new work of this type to the appropriate section based on the description below.

Original Articles may describe research studies of any type or design. The section is appropriate for articles describing methodologically rigorous studies and studies that generate complex results. Articles that describe clinical trials should generally comport with the Consolidated Standards of Reporting Trials (CONSORT) Statement and guidelines (see www.consort-statement.org and its links). Clinical trials also must be registered at an accepted online repository before enrollment. Most Phase II and Phase III trials should be registered at either the National Institute of Health site, http://www.clinicaltrials.gov, or the International Standard Randomized Controlled Trials site, http://www.controlled-trials.com (see http://www.clinicaltrials.gov for guidance concerning the types of trials that must be registered). The maximum length for Original Articles is 3500 words (not including Abstract or references) and the text should be divided into sections with the headings Abstract (see below), Introduction, Methods, Results, Discussion, Disclosures and Acknowledgments, and References. In the Methods section of an article describing a clinical trial, please include a statement about where the registration information is available.

Brief Reports may describe research studies of any type or design. The section is appropriate for work that can be described succinctly, often because it is preliminary, largely confirmatory, or limited by its design or methodology. Articles that describe clinical trials should generally comport with the Consolidated Standards of Reporting Trials (CONSORT) Statement and guidelines (see www.consort-statement.org and its links). Clinical trials also must be registered at an accepted online repository before enrollment. The maximum length of a Brief Report is 2500 words (not including Abstract or references) and the text should be divided into sections with the headings Abstract (see below), Introduction, Methods, Results, Discussion, Disclosures and Acknowledgments, and References.

Brief Methodological Reports present research studies that are intended to expand the measurement capabilities of existing instruments. Although translation may be part of the reported work, appropriate submissions typically describe validation or statistical innovation. The maximum length is 2500 words (not including Abstract or references) and the text should be divided into sections with the headings Abstract (see below), Introduction, Methods, Results, Discussion, Disclosures and Acknowledgments, and References.

Brief Quality Improvement Reports present quality improvement research. Appropriate submissions describe the problem that has been addressed, the quality framework used to implement change, and the specific methods and outcomes. Details sufficient to encourage replication are encouraged. The maximum length is 2500 words (not including Abstract or references) and an Abstract is required (see below). Suggested headings include Background, Measures, Intervention, Outcomes, Conclusions/ Lessons Learned.

Clinical Notes are case series or small observational studies describing new or interesting clinical observations. The maximum length is 2500 words (not including Abstract or references) and an Abstract is required (is required). Suggested headings include Introduction, Methods, Results, Discussion, Disclosures and Acknowledgments, and References.

Palliative Care Rounds couple a case description that includes an important clinical observation with a brief narrative review that discusses the evidence surrounding the observation or best clinical practices related to assessment and management. The specific objective of this section is to provide case-based information relevant to the clinical practice of palliative care. The maximum length is

2500 words (not including Abstract or references) and an Abstract is not required. Suggested headings include Introduction, Case Description, Discussion, Disclosures and Acknowledgments, andReferences.

Letters may be used to report case descriptions or preliminary observations acquired through studies. They are also a forum for opinion, including specific comments related to a previously published article. Letters may undergo external review, and those that comment on a prior *JPSM* publication are typically forwarded to the authors of this publication for a response. Letters are published online only; the title and a link to the *JPSM* website appears in the contents of the printed Journal. The maximum length for all types of Letters is 1250 words (not including references); no more than 10 references and one table or figure is suggested. Letters should begin with "To the Editor." Those that describe research findings may use additional headings, include Methods, Results, Comment, and References; those that present a case description may include the headings Case Description, Comment, and References.

Note: JPSM publishes clinical observations, experiences and reviews of existing work in multiple sections. Please submit new work of this type to the appropriate section based on the description below.

Reviews describe and evaluate previously published material. The emphasis is on systematic reviews, but high-quality narrative reviews will be considered. Systematic reviews should comport with the minimum standards described in the Preferred Reporting Items for Systematic Reviews and Meta-Analyses (www.prisma-statement.org) or comparable guideline. The maximum length of a Review is 7000 words and an Abstract is required (see below).

Special Articles and Special Series Articles JPSM may consider an article that does not fit into other sections as a Special Article. In some cases, a thematically-linked group of these articles is developed as a Special Series on behalf of an organization or through the efforts of an individual. Topics have included program descriptions, meeting proceedings, calls for research, new hypotheses, and descriptions of understudied or poorly recognized areas of clinical interest. The maximum length of a Special Article is 7000 words and an Abstract is required (see below).

Note: JPSM publishes reports that focus on specific areas or interests, as described below. Please submit new work to the appropriate section.

Ethical Issues in Palliative Care couple a case description that includes an observation or experience with important ethical implications to a brief narrative review that provides a bioethical analysis. The maximum length is 2500 words (not including Abstract or references) and an Abstract is not required. Suggested headings include Introduction, Case Description, Defining Issues and Ethical Analysis, Conclusion of the Case, Comment, and References.

Humanities: Art, Language, and Spirituality in Health presents experiences and observations that epitomize the humanistic concerns and challenges encountered in the care of seriously ill patients and their families. Articles may be case descriptions or personal accounts. The maximum length is 2500 words and an Abstract is not required. Authors interested in submitting work to this section are strongly encouraged to write the Managing Editor to indicate this interest and describe the planned submission. Feedback about the proposed submission will be provided by an Editor of this section.

Therapeutic Reviews present and critically evaluate the use of specific drugs and drug classes used in palliative care. This section represents an ongoing collaboration between *JPSM* and the Editors of www.palliativedrugs.com, at which additional content is provided. Authors interested in submitting similar content should consider other sections of JPSM, including Reviews or Special Articles.

Educational Exchange describes innovations related to pedagogy in palliative care. The maximum length is 2500 words and an Abstract is not required. Authors interested in submitting work to this section are strongly encouraged to write the Managing Editor to indicate this interest and describe the planned submission. Feedback about the proposed submission will be provided by an Editor of this section.

Media Reviews Books, monographs, films, and other materials submitted for review should be sent to the editorial office of the Journal, c/o David Newcombe, *Journal of Pain and Symptom Management*, 20 North Street, Plymouth, MA 02360, USA.

Manuscript Submission

The *JPSM* uses a web-based online manuscript submission and review system. Please go to https://www.editorialmanager.com/JPSM/default.aspx to submit your manuscript electronically. The website guides authors stepwise through the creation and uploading of the various files.

All correspondence, including the Editor's decision and request for revisions, will be by e-mail. Authors may send queries concerning the submission process, manuscript status, or journal procedures to the Editorial Office at JPSM@Stellarmed.com.

Submission checklist

You can use this list to carry out a final check of your submission before you send it to the journal for review. Please check the relevant section in this Guide for Authors for more details.

Ensure that the following items are present:

One author has been designated as the corresponding author with contact details:

- E-mail address
- Full postal address

All necessary files have been uploaded:

Manuscript:

- Include keywords
- All figures (include relevant captions)
- All tables (including titles, description, footnotes)
- Ensure all figure and table citations in the text match the files provided
- Indicate clearly if color should be used for any figures in

print *Graphical Abstracts / Highlights files* (where applicable)
Supplemental files (where applicable)

Further considerations

- Manuscript has been 'spell checked' and 'grammar checked'
- All references mentioned in the Reference List are cited in the text, and viceversa
- Permission has been obtained for use of copyrighted material from other sources (including the Internet)
- A competing interests statement is provided, even if the authors have no competing interests to declare
- Journal policies detailed in this guide have been reviewed
- Referee suggestions and contact details provided, based on journal requirements

For further information, visit our Support Center.

Before you begin

Ethics in publishing

Please see our information pages on Ethics in publishing and Ethical guidelines for journal publication.

Conflict of interest

All authors MUST disclose any financial and personal relationships with other people or organizations that could inappropriately influence (bias) their work. Examples of potential conflicts of interest include employment, consultancies, stock ownership, honoraria, paid expert testimony, patent applications/registrations, and grants or other funding. A conflict of interest form is integrated into the submission process and must be completed before your submission is finalized. See also

Submission declaration

Submission of an article implies that the work described has not been published previously (except in the form of an abstract or as part of a published lecture or academic book or as an electronic preprint, that it is not under consideration for publication elsewhere, that its publication is approved by all authors and tacitly or explicitly by the responsible authorities where the work was carried out, and that, if accepted, it will not be published elsewhere including electronically in the same form, in English or in any other language, without the written consent of the copyright-holder. This information may be included in the cover letter.

Use of inclusive language

Inclusive language acknowledges diversity, conveys respect to all people, is sensitive to differences, and promotes equal opportunities. Articles should make no assumptions about the beliefs or commitments of any reader, should contain nothing which might imply that one individual is superior to another on the grounds of race, sex, culture or any other characteristic, and should use inclusive language throughout. Authors should ensure that writing is free from bias, for instance by using 'he or she', 'his/her' instead of 'he' or 'his', and by making use of job titles that are free of stereotyping (e.g. 'chairperson' instead of 'chairman' and 'flight attendant' instead of 'stewardess').

Copyright

Upon acceptance of an article, authors will be asked to complete a 'Journal Publishing Agreement' (see more information on this). An e-mail will be sent to the corresponding author confirming receipt of the manuscript together with a 'Journal Publishing Agreement' form or a link to the online version of this agreement.

Subscribers may reproduce tables of contents or prepare lists of articles including abstracts for internal circulation within their institutions. Permission of the Publisher is required for resale or distribution outside the institution and for all other derivative works, including compilations and translations. If excerpts from other copyrighted works are included, the author(s) must obtain written permission from the copyright owners and credit the source(s) in the article. Elsevier has preprinted forms for use by authors in these cases.

For gold open access articles: Upon acceptance of an article, authors will be asked to complete an 'Exclusive License Agreement' (more information). Permitted third party reuse of gold open access articles is determined by the author's choice of user license.

Author rights

As an author you (or your employer or institution) have certain rights to reuse your work. More information.

Manuscripts should be submitted exclusively to the *Journal of Pain and Symptom Management*. Manuscripts are reviewed and edited with the understanding that the authors are transferring all copyright ownership to the American Academy of Hospice and Palliative Medicine.

Elsevier supports responsible sharing

Find out how you can share your research published in Elsevier journals.

Role of the funding source

You are requested to identify who provided financial support for the conduct of the research and/or preparation of the article and to briefly describe the role of the sponsor(s), if any, in study design; in the collection, analysis and interpretation of data; in the writing of the report; and in the decision to submit the article for publication. If the funding source(s) had no such involvement then this should be stated.

Open access

Please visit our Open Access page for more information.

Language (usage and editing services)

Manuscripts should be written in proper English (American or British usage is accepted, but not a mixture of these). Authors who feel their English language manuscript may require editing to eliminate possible grammatical or spelling errors and to conform to correct scientific English may wish to use the English Language Editing service available from Elsevier's WebShop http://webshop.elsevier.com/languageediting/ or visit our customer support site https://service.elsevier.com for more information.

Confidentiality/Informed Consent/IRB or Ethics Committee Review

It is the author's responsibility to ensure patient anonymity in case reports and elsewhere. Identifying information such as names, initials, hospital numbers, and dates must be avoided. Reports of studies involving human subjects must include a statement verifying:

1) that all patients/other paticipants provided written informed consent or that an institutional review board/ethics committee determined that informed consent was not required; and 2) the study was approved by the investigator's institutional review board/ethics committee.

Submission

Our online submission system guides you stepwise through the process of entering your article details and uploading your files. The system converts your article files to a single PDF file used in the peer-review process. Editable files (e.g., Word, LaTeX) are required to typeset your article for final publication. All correspondence, including notification of the Editor's decision and requests for revision, is sent by e-mail.

Clinical Trial Registration

JPSM requires that human clinical trials are registered before enrollment in order for the results to be published in the journal. Most Phase II and Phase III trials should be registered at either the National Institute of Health site at http://www.clinicaltrials.gov, the International Standard Randomized Controlled Trials site at http://www.controlled-trials.com, or an equivalent national site for public reporting of trials. For questions about the requirement to register at http://www.clinicaltrials.gov, please consult the Checklist and Elaboration for Evaluating Whether a Clinical Trial or Study is an

Applicable Clinical Trial, which is available on the site. The Methods section of the paper reporting the results of a clinical trial should contain a statement about where the registration information is available to the public.

Submit your article

Please submit your article via https://www.editorialmanager.com/JPSM/default.aspx.

Peer Review

Manuscripts submitted to the *Journal of Pain and Symptom Management* undergo initial editorial review. Selected manuscripts are sent for external peer review. Note that reviewers are not blinded as to the author's identity.

Manuscript Preparation

Submission items include a cover letter and all elements of the manuscript (including title page, key words, running title, manuscript text, disclosures and acknowledgments, references, tables and figures). Complete instructions for electronic artwork submission can be found at www.elsevier.com/artwork.

Preparing Electronic Files

Text and graphics may be submitted as separate files in the following formats:

Text: Use Microsoft Word, WordPerfect, WordPro or Rich Text Format (.rtf). Check the accuracy of all file conversions.

Graphics: Create digital artwork after consulting the Artwork and media instructions page, which contains appropriate instructions. Please note that Elsevier allows the submission of MS Office files (Word, PowerPoint, Excel) provided that they meet certain criteria (see information given on Electronic Artwork website). It is preferred to save files in JPEG or TIFF format. Label figures as referenced in text and include a list of figure legends.

Essential title page information

The title page must include: all authors' full first and last names, degrees, and current institutional affiliations, cities and countries; the name, address, and e-mail address of the designated corresponding author; and a list of the number of tables, figures, and references and the word count for the submission.

Abstract, Key Message, Key Words, and Running Title

Abstract: A concise, ***structured*** abstract of not more than 250 words is required for Original Articles, Review Articles, Brief Reports, and Brief Methodological Reports. The abstract should have the following headings: Context, Objectives, Methods, Results, and Conclusion. For Clinical Notes, Palliative Care Rounds, Ethical Issues in Palliative Care, and Special Articles, the Journal will accept either a structured or narrative abstract of no more than 250 words. For Brief Quality Improvement Reports, a *structured* abstract of no more than 150 words is required; headings are: Background, Measures, Intervention, Outcomes, Conclusions/Lessons Learned. Letters should not have abstracts. Abstracts should be on a separate page and follow the title page.*Key Message*: Between the Abstract and the Introduction, we strongly suggest including a *Key Message* statement. This statement, limited to 50 words, should synopsize the work and highlight its significance. Example:

Key Message: This article describes a prospective cohort study that describes the prevalence of breathlessness in a previously unstudied population--patients with The results

indicate that the symptom is highly prevalent, worsens over time, and leads to functional impairment that may be amenable to better symptom control." References should not be included in this *Key Message.*

Key Words: Immediately after the abstract, please provide a maximum of 6 key words, using American spelling and avoiding general and plural terms and multiple concepts (avoid, for example, 'and', 'of'). Be sparing with abbreviations: only abbreviations firmly established in the field may be eligible. These key words will be used for indexing purposes.

Running Title: Please provide a running title of no more than 45 characters and spaces.

NOTE: Abstracts, key words and running title must be included with the Word document of the submission, not just provided online.

Disclosures and Acknowledgments

For ALL types of manuscript submissions, except Letters, authors must complete the ICMJE Form for Disclosure of Potential Conflicts of Interest, which can be found here: http://www.icmje.org/conflicts-of-interest/. In addition, a Disclosure/Conflict of Interest section should be placed after the text and before the References. It must include a disclosure/conflict of interest statement that refers to all the authors. Please either indicate the lack of conflict (i.e., nothing to disclose) or list possible conflicts for each named author. The statement should be consistent with the ICMJE form. Conflicts of Interest include financial or other relationships that could be perceived to influence the manuscript. If uncertain as to what might be considered a potential conflict of interest, authors should err on the side of full disclosure. An Acknowledgments section, if included, should be placed after the Disclosure/Conflict of Interest section, just before the references. It may include the authors' expressions of gratitude, including mention of individuals who contributed to the work but whose involvement was not sufficient to warrant authorship.

Formatting of funding sources

List funding sources in this standard way to facilitate compliance to funder's requirements:

Funding: This work was supported by the National Institutes of Health [grant numbers xxxx, yyyy]; the Bill & Melinda Gates Foundation, Seattle, WA [grant number zzzz]; and the United States Institutes of Peace [grant number aaaa].

It is not necessary to include detailed descriptions on the program or type of grants and awards. When funding is from a block grant or other resources available to a university, college, or other research institution, submit the name of the institute or organization that provided the funding.

If no funding has been provided for the research, please include the following sentence:

This research did not receive any specific grant from funding agencies in the public, commercial, or not-for-profit sectors.

Units

Follow internationally accepted rules and conventions: use the international system of units (SI). If other units are mentioned, please give their equivalent in SI.

Artwork Illustrations

Black-and-white photographs or line drawings are preferred. Separate typed legends should accompany each figure. Every figure must be cited in the text. If original artwork/photos are used, permission must be obtained from the artist or photographer and credit must be given. If subjects of photographs are persons and they are identifiable, permission must be obtained.

Electronic artwork

General points

- Make sure you use uniform lettering and sizing of your original artwork.
- Embed the used fonts if the application provides that option.
- Aim to use the following fonts in your illustrations: Arial, Courier, Times New Roman, Symbol, or use fonts that look similar.
- Number the illustrations according to their sequence in the text.
- Use a logical naming convention for your artwork files.
- Provide captions to illustrations separately.
- Size the illustrations close to the desired dimensions of the published version.
- Submit each illustration as a separate file.
- Ensure that color images are accessible to all, including those with impaired colorvision.

A detailed guide on electronic artwork is available.

You are urged to visit this site; some excerpts from the detailed information are given here.

Formats

If your electronic artwork is created in a Microsoft Office application (Word, PowerPoint, Excel) then please supply 'as is' in the native document format.

Regardless of the application used other than Microsoft Office, when your electronic artwork is finalized, please 'Save as' or convert the images to one of the following formats (note the resolution requirements for line drawings, halftones, and line/halftone combinations given below):

EPS (or PDF): Vector drawings, embed all used fonts.

TIFF (or JPEG): Color or grayscale photographs (halftones), keep to a minimum of 300 dpi.

TIFF (or JPEG): Bitmapped (pure black & white pixels) line drawings, keep to a minimum of 1000 dpi.
TIFF (or JPEG): Combinations bitmapped line/half-tone (color or grayscale), keep to a minimum of 500 dpi.

Please do not:

- Supply files that are optimized for screen use (e.g., GIF, BMP, PICT, WPG); these typically have a low number of pixels and limited set of colors;
- Supply files that are too low in resolution;
- Submit graphics that are disproportionately large for the content.

Tables

Type each table double-spaced on a separate page, number in order of appearance, and give a brief descriptive title. Every table must be cited in the text. Explanatory information should be placed in footnotes; note that the Journal uses superscript, italic Arabic letters for footnotes, not other symbols, e.g., asterisks. If the data shown are from another source, acknowledgment must be given and permission obtained. **Note: Lengthy tables may be published online only, with a link to the Journal website indicated in the print article text. The determination regarding online publication only will be made by the Editor-in-Chief.**

References

Number references in order of their use in the text; do not alphabetize. Identify references in the text with Arabic numerals inside parentheses. When listing authors in the reference list: Five authors or less, list all five authors; six authors or more, list the first three authors followed by et al. For abbreviations of journal names, refer to *List of Journals Indexed in Index Medicus*. Provide inclusive page numbers. Reference accuracy is the responsibility of the author(s). Please do not use EndNote to compile your reference list.

Examples of Reference Style:

Journal Article

Hatler CW, Grove C, Strickland S, Barron S, White BD. The effect of completing a surrogacy information and decision-making tool upon admission to an intensive care unit on length of stay and charges. J Clin Ethics 2012;23:129-138.

Book Chapter

Taylor C, Walker S. Compassion: luxury or necessity? In: Cobb M, Puchalski CM, Rumbold B, eds. Oxford textbook of spirituality in healthcare. New York: Oxford University Press, 2012:135-144.

Book

Cassell EJ. The nature of suffering and the goals of medicine, 2nd ed. New York: Oxford University Press, 2004.

Online Citations: World Health Organization. Definition of palliative care. 2008. Available from: http://www.who.int/cancer/palliative/ definition/en/. Accessed July 27, 2013.

Citation in text

Please ensure that every reference cited in the text is also present in the reference list (and vice versa). Any references cited in the abstract must be given in full. Unpublished results and personal communications are not recommended in the reference list, but may be mentioned in the text. If these references are included in the reference list they should follow the standard reference style of the journal and should include a substitution of the publication date with either 'Unpublished results' or 'Personal communication'. Citation of a reference as 'in press' implies that the item has been accepted for publication.

Reference links

Increased discoverability of research and high quality peer review are ensured by online links to the sources cited. In order to allow us to create links to abstracting and indexing services, such as Scopus, CrossRef and PubMed, please ensure that data provided in the references are correct. Please note that incorrect surnames, journal/book titles, publication year and pagination may prevent link creation. When copying references, please be careful as they may already contain errors. Use of the DOI is highly encouraged.

A DOI is guaranteed never to change, so you can use it as a permanent link to any electronic article. An example of a citation using DOI for an article not yet in an issue is: VanDecar J.C., Russo R.M., James D.E., Ambeh W.B., Franke M. (2003). Aseismic continuation of the Lesser Antilles slab beneath northeastern Venezuela. Journal of Geophysical Research, https://doi.org/10.1029/2001JB000884. Please note the format of such citations should be in the same style as all other references in the paper.

Data references

This journal encourages you to cite underlying or relevant datasets in your manuscript by citing them in your text and including a data reference in your Reference List. Data references should include the following elements: author name(s), dataset title, data repository, version (where available), year, and global persistent identifier. Add [dataset] immediately before the reference so we can properly identify it as a data reference. The [dataset] identifier will not appear in your published article.

Journal abbreviations source

Journal names should be abbreviated according to the List of Title Word Abbreviations.

Research data

This journal encourages and enables you to share data that supports your research publication where appropriate, and enables you to interlink the data with your published articles. Research data refers to the results of observations or experimentation that validate research findings. To facilitate reproducibility and data reuse, this journal also encourages you to share your software, code, models, algorithms, protocols, methods and other useful materials related to the project.

Below are a number of ways in which you can associate data with your article or make a statement about the availability of your data when submitting your manuscript. If you are sharing data in one of these ways, you are encouraged to cite the data in your manuscript and reference list. Please refer to the "References" section for more information about data citation. For more information on depositing, sharing and using research data and other relevant research materials, visit the research data page.

Data linking

If you have made your research data available in a data repository, you can link your article directly to the dataset. Elsevier collaborates with a number of repositories to link articles on ScienceDirect with relevant repositories, giving readers access to underlying data that gives them a better understanding of the research described.

There are different ways to link your datasets to your article. When available, you can directly link your dataset to your article by providing the relevant information in the submission system. For more information, visit the database linking page.

For supported data repositories a repository banner will automatically appear next to your published article on ScienceDirect.In addition, you can link to relevant data or entities through identifiers within the text of your manuscript, using the following format: Database: xxxx (e.g., TAIR: AT1G01020; CCDC: 734053; PDB: 1XFN).

Mendeley Data

This journal supports Mendeley Data, enabling you to deposit any research data (including raw and processed data, video, code, software, algorithms, protocols, and methods) associated with your manuscript in a free-to-use, open access repository. During the submission process, after uploading your manuscript, you will have the opportunity to upload your relevant datasets directly to *Mendeley Data*. The datasets will be listed and directly accessible to readers next to your published article online.

For more information, visit the Mendeley Data for journals page.

Data statement

To foster transparency, we encourage you to state the availability of your data in your submission. This may be a requirement of your funding body or institution. If your data is unavailable to access or unsuitable to post, you will have the opportunity to indicate why during the submission process, for example by stating that the research data is confidential. The statement will appear with your published article on ScienceDirect. For more information, visit the Data Statement page.

After Acceptance

Proofs

One set of page proofs (as PDF files) will be sent by e-mail to the corresponding author. Elsevier now provides authors with PDF proofs which can be annotated; for this you will need to download Adobe Reader version 7 (or higher) available free from http://get.adobe.com/reader. Instructions on how to annotate PDF files will accompany the proofs (also given online). The exact system requirements are given at the Adobe site: http://www.adobe.com/products/reader/tech-specs.html.

If you do not wish to use the PDF annotations function, you may list the corrections (including replies to the Query Form) and return them to Elsevier in an e-mail. Please list your corrections quoting line number. If, for any reason, this is not possible, then mark the corrections and any other comments (including replies to the Query Form) on a printout of your proof and return by fax, or scan the pages and e-mail. Please use this proof only for checking the typesetting, editing, completeness and correctness of the text, tables and figures. Significant changes to the article as accepted for publication will only be considered at this stage with permission from the Editor. We will do everything possible to get your article published quickly and accurately – please let us have all your corrections within 48 hours. It is important to ensure that all corrections are sent back to us in one communication: please check carefully before replying, as inclusion of any subsequent corrections cannot be guaranteed. Proofreading is solely your responsibility. Note that Elsevier may proceed with the publication of your article if no response is received.

Offprints

The corresponding author will, at no cost, receive a customized Share Link providing 50 days free access to the final published version of the article on ScienceDirect. The Share Link can be used for sharing the article via any communication channel, including email and social media. For an extra charge, paper offprints can be ordered via the offprint order form which is sent once the article is accepted for publication. Both corresponding and co-authors may order offprints at any time via Elsevier's Author Services. Corresponding authors who have published their article gold open access do not receive a Share Link as their final published version of the article is available open access on ScienceDirect and can be shared through the article DOI link.

Note to NIH Grant Recipients

Elsevier will send to PubMed Central the author's manuscript on behalf of authors reporting research supported by an NIH grant. The author manuscript reflects any author-agreed changes made in response to peer review comments. Elsevier will authorize its public access posting on PubMed Central 12 months after final publication. Authors will receive further correspondence from PubMed Central after the manuscript is deposited.

Author Inquiries

Visit the Elsevier Support Center to find the answers you need. Here you will find everything from Frequently Asked Questions to ways to get in touch.

You can also check the status of your submitted article or find out when your accepted article will be published

www.ingramcontent.com/pod-product-compliance
Lightning Source LLC
LaVergne TN
LVHW041129150826
845673LV00007B/2236

9783384266545